Baby Tips

Pregnancy Tips for Moms-to-Be

Baby Tips®

Pregnancy Tips for Moms-to-Be

Karen N. Salt

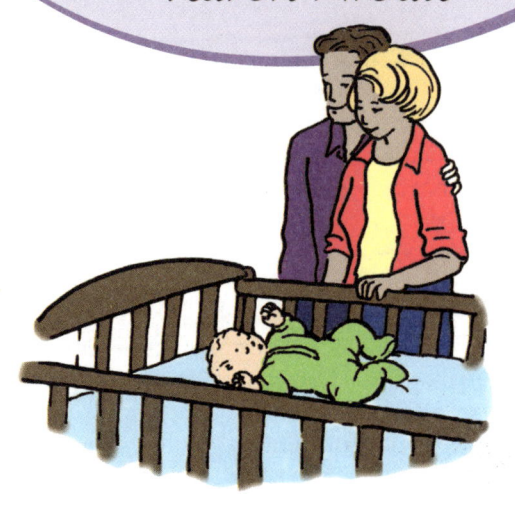

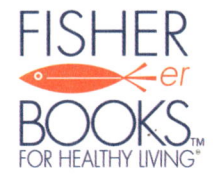

FISHER
BOOKS™
FOR HEALTHY LIVING®

Publishers:	Howard W. Fisher
	Helen V. Fisher
Managing Editor:	Sarah Trotta
Illustrations:	Cathie Lowmiller
Book design & production:	Randy Schultz
Cover design:	Lynn Bishop
Index:	Michelle Graye

Published by Fisher Books, LLC
5225 W. Massingale Road
Tucson, Arizona 85743-8416
(520) 744-6110
www.fisherbooks.com

Printed in U.S.A.

10 9 8 7 6 5 4 3 2 1

Note: The information in this book is true and complete to the best of our knowledge. This book is intended only as an informative guide for those wishing to know more about pregnancy. In no way is this book intended to replace, countermand or conflict with the advice given to you by your physician. The information in this book is general and is offered with no guarantees on the part of the author or Fisher Books. The author and publisher disclaim all liability in connection with the use of this book.

Contents

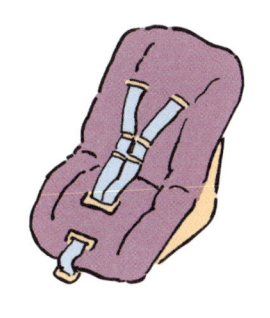

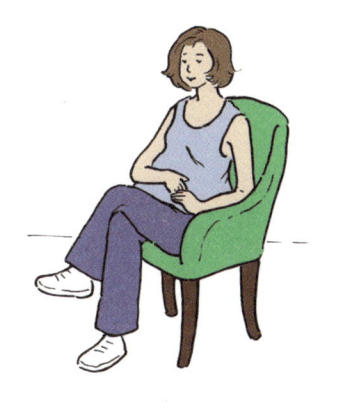

Introduction

If you just found out that you are pregnant, let me offer my congratulations. I promise not to hound you about the baby's sex, potential name, or your due date. Happy reading!

I'll bet you can't believe it . . . you are going to be a mother. Are you excited? Nervous? Maybe just a little anxious? Don't be! This book will help. While no one can promise to make everything go perfectly, *Pregnancy Tips for Moms-to-Be* does offer you the kind of pregnancy support, guidance and information that I think every mom-to-be needs. But don't stop here. Talk to other new moms, your family members and your healthcare providers. Check out other resources too (many are suggested for you at the end of this book). Your baby needs you to be as prepared as possible. Are you? All you need to do is turn the page . . .

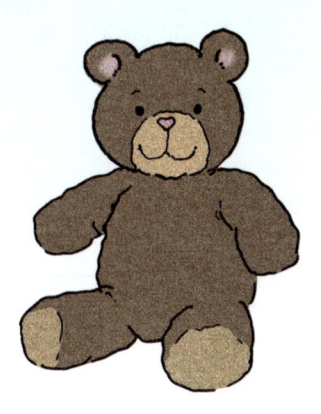

Physical Changes and Stages

Admit it: Most of us think we're pregnant when our cycles fail to start exactly on time. This usually doesn't mean much because our period often starts a couple of days later, as soon as our stress level goes down. But sometimes . . . days turn into weeks. And bingo!

Your breasts become heavy. The bathroom becomes your new friend. And your eyes close in seconds before sleep. Welcome to pregnancy!

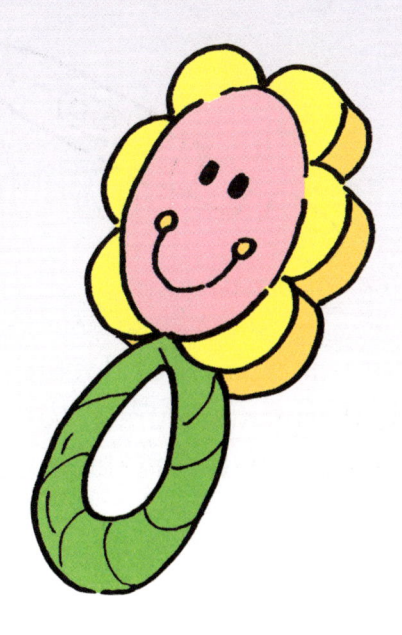

You need to be a number of weeks into your pregnancy before most over-the-counter pregnancy tests are considered accurate.

A hormone called *human chorionic gonadotropin* is measured in all urine-based pregnancy tests available over-the-counter from most drug stores.

Even if you have taken an over-the-counter pregnancy test, your practitioner will still want to take a sample of your blood to confirm or deny that you are pregnant.

A blood test done at your doctor's or midwife's office is the most accurate way to check for pregnancy, especially during the early weeks.

Prenatal Appointments and You

Many of the tips listed in this section touch on subjects that are discussed and explained by most doctors and midwives at any of your many, many prenatal appointments. You owe it to yourself and your baby to go to all of these visits, not because pregnancy and birth are particularly risky, but because you should monitor your health and your baby's at this time just to be safe.

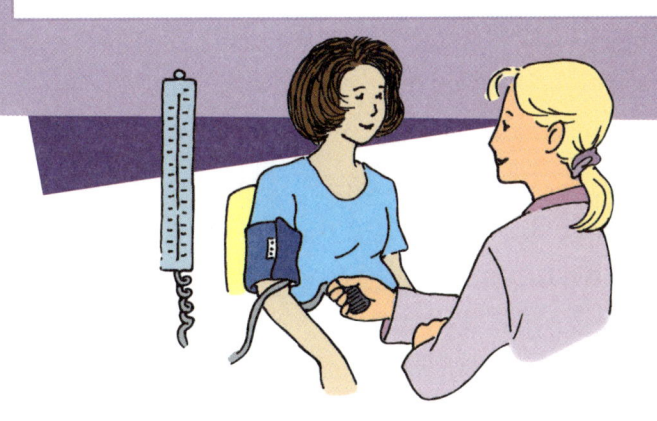

Early pregnancy changes make breasts tender and urination frequent. These uncomfortable changes are normal. They may challenge your sense of humor sometimes, but they will lessen as pregnancy advances, only to make a repeat appearance during the last few months.

Fatigue and morning sickness are common early pregnancy discomforts moms mention. For most women, these conditions lessen around 13 weeks of pregnancy.

Tired?

Your body is going through great changes, from pumping extra blood throughout your body to growing a new life—no wonder you feel tired! Take care of yourself! Rest whenever possible. Let go of nonessential activities right now, such as getting the living room extra-clean or staying up until 3:00 A.M. to rearrange the house. The living room and the rest of your house will still be there tomorrow.

If you work outside the home and it's hard to schedule a naptime, use your lunchtime or other break to rest for 20 or 30 minutes. Prop up your feet, close your eyes and sit in a quiet spot. Think about something soothing and restful, such as imagining the lapping of waves on a beach, or the flicker of a single candle flame in a dark room.

Most doctors and midwives will talk about your pregnancy being in a certain week of development, rather than a certain month. It's more precise that way.

Even though we talk about being "nine months pregnant"—which should be 270 days, or 36 weeks—practitioners add almost 3 extra weeks to that figure, starting from the first day of the last menstrual cycle. They do this to account for the baby's initial gestation period. That brings the length of the pregnancy up to 40 weeks, the time that a pregnacy is considered full-term.

Being pregnant for three months means that you have ended your 12th week, finished your first trimester, and hopefully put any bouts of morning sickness behind you!

During weeks 9 to 12 of your pregnancy, you probably will have the option at a prenatal visit of hearing your baby's heartbeat with a hand-held Doppler ultrasound device. It is a relatively safe procedure, but it *is* an option—you should feel comfortable with having it done. If you don't want to do it, you don't have to.

Few moments are as special as the first time you hear your baby's heartbeat.

If you choose to hear your baby's heartbeat at an early prenatal visit, bring along a tape recorder to capture it for yourself and others (such as Grandma).

During the first trimester, it's a good idea to purchase pants, skirts and dresses one or two sizes larger than you normally wear. These clothes will give you a little growing room in the months ahead.

Even though you are not showing at 3 months, you are probably feeling fuller than usual. Unfortunately, you're still too small for maternity wear, but too big for your normal clothes. You might try borrowing your man's larger shirts to wear over comfortable leggings. That's just one idea. The point is to look good and feel comfortable.

You may not experience any fatigue or morning sickness during the first few months of your pregnancy. Instead, you may have what can only be called "that glow." You skin shimmers and shines. Your hair falls in cascading waves for the first time in your life. You aren't moaning about anything, honey. You—mommy—are healthy, vibrant and strong!

Oooh ... I Don't Feel Well

Morning sickness, which can happen at any time of day, is not fun. But you can do certain things that may help relieve the nausea you feel.

- ✿ Don't let yourself get too hungry—an empty stomach is a recipe for morning sickness. (In fact, for this reason it's a good idea to nibble a few plain crackers before you get out of bed in the morning.) Keep saltine crackers handy for snacking. Slices of tart apples work for some women.
- ✿ Drink plenty of fluids throughout the day, especially water; you can also drink juice, lemonade, or fruit tea, milk or carbonated drinks, if you like them.
- ✿ Sipping ginger tea helps many women overcome a sudden feeling of nausea.
- ✿ Other women get relief by using anti-nausea wristbands, which put pressure on the inside of the wrist. These wristbands were developed originally as an effective remedy for seasickness.

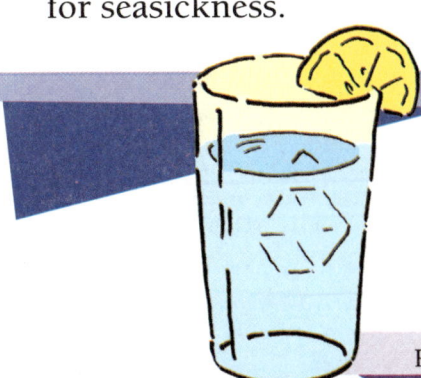

1ST Trimester

Don't get excited if you notice changes in your skin. It is simply responding, like the rest of you, to the hormones of pregnancy.

If your skin changes from flaky to oily or dry to combination, don't fret—simply clean, as needed, and keep going.

You can't do anything about color changes to your skin, though. Think of the new freckles or dark pigment as a sign of motherhood.

1ST Trimester

You have probably already noticed one change right under your nose—your breasts. Most women feel changes in their breasts immediately. Because extra blood is flowing into the breasts in preparation for milk production, they tend to feel heavy and full (as they can during ovulation). All of your breast tissue is stimulated to prepare to feed a baby. Instead of enlarging and then shrinking back to size, your breasts will continue to grow.

1ST Trimester

Your baby boy at 12 weeks gestation has all of his organs, although they are small and not fully developed. This is extraordinary growth. From a cluster of cells, he is already a baby. And here is the most surprising part: Your baby is still only about 3 inches long!

Imagine your baby inside of you at 12 weeks! Make sure you imagine her opening her mouth, and opening and closing her hands. She can do all of these things, even at this young age.

Over-the-Counter Medications

Most of us are comfortable popping an aspirin or drinking a teaspoon of cough syrup, obtained from the aisles of our local drug store, when we're not feeling well.

While many of these OTCs (over-the-counter medications) are safe during pregnancy, others definitely are not! Certain cough syrups contain caffeine and codeine substitutes. Other medications contain substances that cause unwanted effects. For example, aspirin contains a compound that may cause excessive bleeding during birth.

My advice: Talk to your doctor or midwife about OTCs. Ask them what they feel is safe *before* you take anything.

2ND Trimester **H**ello beautiful mama of the sixth-month belly. Your baby is about 12 inches long now and you can feel *all* of her.

2ND Trimester **C**ongratulations! Now that you have carried your baby for 21 to 25 weeks, you have crossed a major threshold: You are more than halfway done with your pregnancy!

2ND Trimester **S**omewhere around week 18, your baby girl starts growing her first lock of hair.

2ND Trimester **N**ow that you are big-bellied and beautiful, you've got to think about resting and keeping yourself comfortable. Having varicose veins or edema (fluid in your tissues) is not comfortable. If you find yourself on your feet all day, try wearing flat shoes *and* resting one foot on a low stool or footrest. (Alternate feet about every 30 minutes.) This trick will help decrease water retention and increase blood circulation.

2ND Trimester One day while walking, you may notice your stomach feels hard, like the outside of a watermelon. This sensation doesn't last too long and it isn't harmful, but it can make bending a little difficult.

2ND Trimester Any brief tightenings in your uterus around your sixth month of pregnancy are usually what's known as *Braxton Hicks contractions*. Mr. Braxton Hicks was not a woman, so he never actually felt these contractions. Someone decided to name these sensations after him because he was the first to describe them in the medical world.

2ND Trimester Any mother will tell you that the Braxton Hicks contractions, or what I call *practice contractions*, in the middle months of pregnancy are neither painful nor frequent.

The frequency with which you experience them will change toward the end of pregnancy, however. That means your body is gearing up for the big day: baby's birth.

3RD Trimester

One thing that certainly changes during the last trimester (months 7 to 9) is sleep. You just can't seem to get comfortable!

You might try sleeping with a body pillow. They can be twisted and stuck in all the right places for comfort and body support: for example, under your tummy and between your knees.

3RD Trimester

Most of us busy women drive. That means we also drive during pregnancy. This isn't a problem unless you feel it is. However, you will want to do two things as your pregnancy advances.

1. Move your lap seat belt under your belly.
2. Move the driver's seat far enough away from the steering wheel that your belly does not touch it.

3RD Trimester

Traveling by air becomes harder and harder once you enter the last few months of pregnancy. This is primarily due to the fact that most airline companies would rather babies not be born on a flight from Los Angeles to Honolulu (or anywhere else mid-air).

3RD Trimester

If you feel compelled to travel during the last few weeks of your pregnancy, make sure that you check with your practitioner *first*. If everything is okay and you can make the trip, you will need to take copies of your medical records with you, just in case. If you are going somewhere for an extended trip (weeks or months), find a practitioner in your destination area to see you until you return home.

3RD Trimester

Once you've reached weeks 26 to 29, it's hard to focus on anything but baby's eminent arrival, and no wonder. He or she seems everywhere inside you—twisting and turning somersaults just for you.

3RD Trimester

Some tasks are harder to do in the last trimester—like tying the shoelaces on a pair of sneakers. There's so much tummy there that you just can't reach your feet. Necessity is the mother of invention, Mom. Improvise! Use steps or boxes to bring your feet closer to your hands.

3RD Trimester — No one wants to have preterm labor, but it can happen. Learn the signs and you'll be prepared, just in case.

Preterm Labor Warning Signs

Let your doctor or midwife know immediately if you experience any of these symptoms.

1. any vaginal bleeding, especially bleeding that is brownish-reddish in color, heavy (like a period), or accompanied by pain in your abdomen

2. sharp pains in your belly or vagina

3. sudden or continuous gushing of clear or colored liquid from your vagina

4. frequent contractions (about 7 to 10) that last for more than an hour

There are other, less obvious preterm labor signs, but these are some of the most critical to look out for.

3RD Trimester — Signs of trouble that you should report to your doctor or midwife immediately include headaches, blurry vision, and swelling in your hands or feet. These are all possible indicators of conditions such as pre-eclampsia or pregnancy-induced high blood pressure that may need monitoring or treatment. Always report any changes in your body to your doctor or midwife, no matter how small.

3RD Trimester — Your baby, who at 29 weeks can see, hear, smell, and taste, weighs more than 2 pounds. She is about 14 inches long at this time.

3RD Trimester — By the time your baby is ready to be born (and only babies know when they are ready), he will weigh, on average, 7-1/2 pounds.

Some women start to feel intense backaches during the last trimester. This could happen for lots of reasons, but one of the most common causes is separated abdominal muscles. Talk to your practitioner if you suspect this may describe your condition.

Separated abdominal muscles have essentially "unzipped" themselves from the place in the body to which they had been attached. In some cases, this happens because of the large size of the uterus (as in a multiple pregnancy). Other cases occur because mom starts pregnancy with weak muscles that cannot take the pressure of the growing uterus.

You can help support separated or weak muscles in your abdomen or lower back by wearing a prenatal support belt or leotard. These products are designed specifically to cradle the uterus and help all of your muscles work together without strain. Check with your doctor or midwife for places to pick one up locally.

3RD Trimester

Don't be surprised when you wake up at 2:00 A.M. the day before your due date with a sudden urge to mop the kitchen floor. This nesting instinct—to clean everything before the new arrival comes—overtakes even the most untidy new mother.

3RD Trimester

It is extremely important during the last few weeks of pregnancy that you rest and eat well. You will need all of your strength during labor to bring your baby into the world.

❀ Get to bed reasonably early. If you are a determined night owl, read or listen to soothing music while lying comfortably in bed until you are sleepy enough to close your eyes.

❀ Fortify the nutrition of your favorite recipes by sneaking in extra vegetables.

More Vegetables, Please

It's pretty easy to add fruits and vegetables to your diet. Here are just a few ideas to get you started.

- ❀ Mix in a package of chopped, frozen spinach (cooked and drained beforehand) to a pot of macaroni and cheese just before serving.

- ❀ Add broccoli flowerets to a salad for crunch.

- ❀ Mix raisins into your egg salad before making a sandwich.

- ❀ Sprinkle dried cranberries over your morning bowl of cereal. Or defrost frozen peach slices, strawberries or blueberries and sprinkle them on instead.

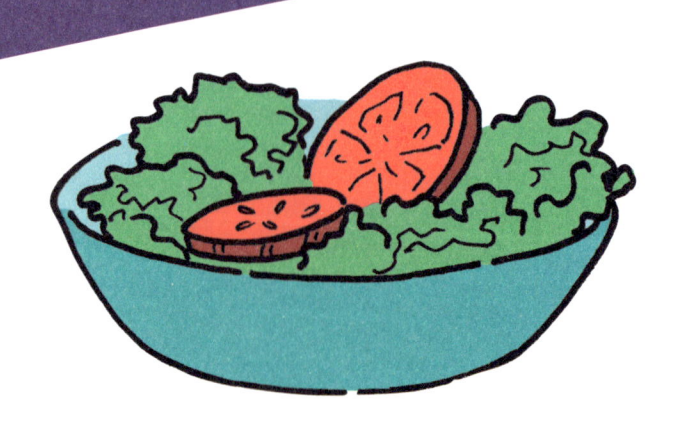

3RD Trimester — Your due date is calculated by counting back 3 months from the first day of your last period, and adding 7 days.

Here's an example: If June 1 was the first day of your last period, subtract 3 months to come up with a March 1 date. Seven days later would be March 8. Your estimated due date would be March 8 of the following year.

3RD Trimester — The reality of your baby's birth day is that it comes when your baby and your body are ready. Lots of women ask their health practitioners about this. The truth is, no magic formula can give you the exact minute of your baby's birth.

3RD Trimester — Your doctor or midwife will come up with one estimated due date based on your last menstrual period. If you have an ultrasound scan, it may provide another date based on your baby's growth. These dates may be different. Instead of feeling confused, feel confident that you have a good idea of your baby's "birth zone."

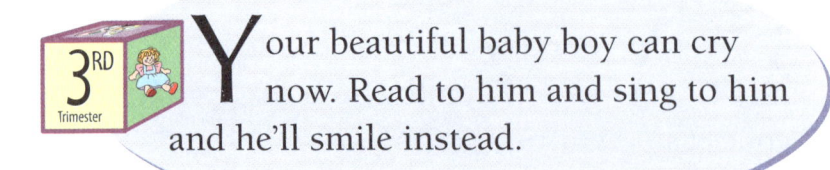

Your beautiful baby boy can cry now. Read to him and sing to him and he'll smile instead.

Your beautiful baby is getting bigger every day. Soon, his somersaults will turn into slower movements. He will eventually settle into his birth position, filling almost every corner of your expanded uterus.

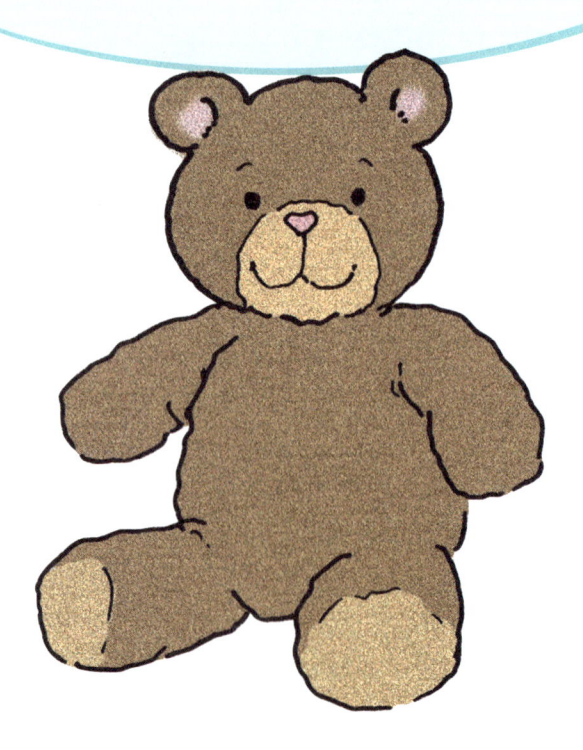

Feeding Body and Soul

A national campaign for better health encourages everyone to eat five to nine servings of fruits and vegetables every day. Find out more about the five-a-day campaign by visiting the http://www.5aday.com web site.

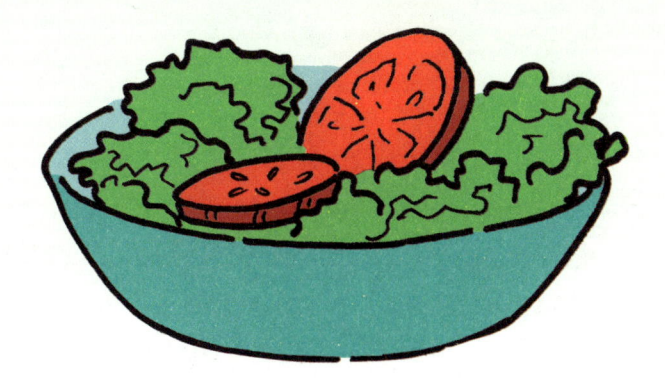

Dedicate yourself to eating well now that you are pregnant. Cut out the junk food such as potato chips and cheeseburgers and treats such as candy bars and sugary cereals. Instead, focus on healthful foods that will help you grow a healthy baby.

It's important that you examine your diet and monitor what you eat to make sure you are getting all of the vitamins, minerals and other nutrients that you and your baby need every day.

Write down what you eat (snacks and all) every day for a week, and take it in to your next prenatal appointment for advice.

For all of you Internet moms . . . check out the Food and Nutrition Information Center of the U.S. Department of Agriculture. This excellent site contains nutritional information, plus an interactive food pyramid to help you create a balanced diet. You can reach this site at http://www.nal.usda.gov/fnic.

Deciding what to eat to attain the Recommended Dietary Allowances (RDAs) for vitamins and minerals takes a certain amount of effort, but it's worthwhile! How tall you are, what you weigh (now and before you were pregnant), what you like to eat and what you can afford all must be factored in. Your doctor, midwife or a registered dietitian can all help you create a balanced menu plan that will include foods you like to eat.

Certain foods when eaten together have a nutritional effect that isn't seen when they are consumed separately. For example, taking iron with orange juice (vitamin C) helps your body absorb the iron better. Without the orange juice, more of the iron will pass through your body and be discarded as a waste product. Eating a fresh spinach salad with fresh orange or tangerine sections tossed in is a terrific way to get more iron!

Recommended Dietary Allowances (RDAs) for Pregnant Women from the Food and Nutrition Board of the National Research Council

The chart that follows reflects the most current RDAs for pregnant women. Remember, your weight, height and body type may change some recommendations for you. Consult your doctor or midwife, or a nutritionist, for specifics, especially if you are a vegetarian or do not eat red meat.

Substance	RDA
Vitamin A	800 micrograms
Vitamin B	10 micrograms
Vitamin K	65 micrograms
Vitamin E	10 milligrams
Vitamin C	70 milligrams
Thiamin	1.5 milligrams
Riboflavin	1.6 milligrams
Niacin	17 milligrams
Vitamin B6	2.2 milligrams
Folate	400 micrograms
Vitamin B12	2.2 micrograms
Calcium	1200 milligrams
Phosphorus	1200 milligrams
Magnesium	320 milligrams
Iron	30 milligrams
Zinc	15 milligrams
Iodine	175 micrograms
Selenium	65 micrograms

Iron and folic acid (folate) are among the many minerals and vitamins that are essential for a pregnant woman to include in her diet. Talk to your practitioner about your diet to make sure you get the recommended daily allowances of all of these good things.

Get 2 for 1

Folic acid and fiber are two of the essential substances that you and your baby need *every day*. Folic acid has been linked to preventing birth defects. Fiber reduces a mom's chances of getting constipated. Now, wouldn't it be great if you could get both things in one food? You can. The following list identifies just a few of the many foods that contain both folic acid *and* fiber. Enjoy them often!

- Avocados
- Broccoli
- Spinach
- Strawberries
- Artichokes
- Blackberries
- Brussels sprouts
- Grapefruit
- Oranges
- Papayas
- Sweet potatoes

It's true: *You are what you eat.* Your baby has tiny organs that are easily overwhelmed by anything besides wholesome food. A baby needs only goodness. Avoid any substances, such as alcohol, and any products, such as cigarettes, that can permanently damage his little body. If you need help quitting *any* substance, talk to your doctor or midwife. There are also support groups in most communities that can supply the much-needed strength to let go of the substance. Alcoholics Anonymous and Nicotine Anonymous are two examples. Both groups have web sites on the Internet as well support groups in thousands of communities.

Every month, almost every women's magazine cover on the newsstands tells readers at least one way to lose weight fast. While I don't suggest that you eat everything in sight just because you're pregnant, I will plead with you *not* to diet. Any yo-yo eating now (lots of food one day, little the next) can stunt your baby's growth and development.

You may have noticed that you can't go as long as you used to between meals. In fact, the longer you wait to eat, the weaker and more nauseated you are likely to become.

To counteract nausea and that awful feeling of fullness after a big meal, spread out your three meals each day to six smaller meals. You'll find it is easier to eat smaller portions more often. This style of eating fights nausea and keeps your energy at a more stable level, too.

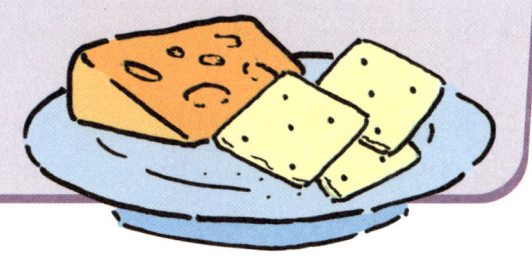

Another way to fight fatigue and hunger during the day is to snack. High-powered snacks such as natural yogurt, fruit and nuts can go a long way toward meeting your nutrition goals. If you are allergic to any of these ideas, don't worry. Simply choose something else that is low in fat and rich in nutrients.

...oothie

...easy to make, and looks and tastes so good.

1 cup natural yogurt
1 or 2 bananas, OR ½ qt. strawberries OR 1 mango, or a combination
5 or 6 ice cubes, approximately
Honey to taste
½ tsp. vanilla extract

Mix yogurt and fruit in a blender. Add ice and continue to blend until ice is crushed. Add honey to taste. Add vanilla extract. Blend briefly to combine all ingredients.

Pour into a tall glass and enjoy! Serves 1.

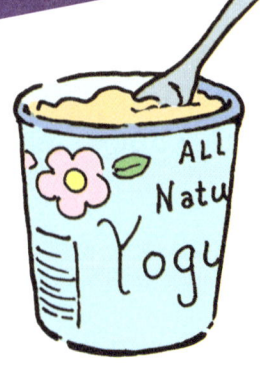

To some people, *exercise* is a foreign word that conjures up images of pounding and sweating to Muzak®. I have a different take on it. I believe that we exercise when we move—it's as simple as that. So walk around the block (or walk around the mall). Try a brisk pace and swing your arms—freely, the way you did when you were seven or eight years old. See how good it makes you feel.

If you are an exercise queen, you can usually continue your activities as long as you don't become overheated. Water-skiing, horseback riding and other high-impact sports or sports requiring good balance probably will be off-limits. Modified aerobics, walking and swimming will probably be fine.

Talk to your practitioner or an exercise physiologist if you need more information about what to do and what to avoid.

Exercise Guidelines for Pregnant Women

Times are changing, my friend. Just 20 years ago, a mother who wanted to exercise during pregnancy was told that she was risking her health.

Welcome to the new millennium. A lot has changed, to you and to the old exercise advice.

The American College of Obstetricians and Gynecologists (ACOG) now feels that exercise during pregnancy is not only safe—as long as there are no health concerns to suggest otherwise—but also is good for us. Studies show that moderate exercise during pregnancy increases baby's weight, and decreases the length of labor and the time of postpartum recovery.

ACOG's current exercise guidelines are outlined briefly here. For more information, talk with your own doctor or midwife.

1. Try to exercise at least three times a week versus taking sporadic exercise every three months. You'll get the most benefit from the exercise if you maintain a steady habit.
2. Try not to exercise when you feel sick.
3. Exercise in comfortable clothes and on surfaces that are lightly carpeted (think "cushioned support").

4. Always warm up properly before and cool down properly after exercising.
5. Monitor your heart rate so that you do not overtax yourself. ACOG recommends staying below 150 beats per minute, especially at peak activity. (Note: Check your heart rate by feeling for your pulse under your chin or along your wrist. Count the beats for 15 seconds against a watch and then multiply by four to equal one minute. That number is your heart rate.)
6. Drink, drink, drink! Take sips of water before, during and after exercising.
7. If you feel any pain or dizziness during your exercise activity, stop immediately. Consult your doctor or midwife.
8. Once your pregnancy is about 20 weeks along, avoid exercises that would require you to lie on your back.

We now know that moderate exercise during pregnancy is good. However, avoid starting a strenuous routine during your pregnancy. The best advice, if you have exercised before, is to do whatever feels good. If you get winded or tired, stop. You can monitor your heart rate, but remember, your resting heart rate will increase as your pregnancy advances.

Some mommies find water exercise and yoga a welcome change to pounding aerobic activity. Check out the recreation centers in your area to see what's available.

One exercise that is essential for you to undertake daily is meditation. While not a physical exercise, meditation is a mental activity that can truly lower your stress and fatigue levels. Check out books and videos from the library and see what regular meditation can do for you.

Meditation Exercise

Done regularly, this practice can help you break a stressed-out mood and help you feel calmer. You can modify this exercise slightly and use it after pregnancy, too.

Sit in a quiet, comfortable place where you won't be disturbed. Dim the lights if possible. Wear comfortable clothing. You may sit on the floor, or in a comfortable chair with your hands in your lap. Breathe slowly and close your eyes.

Focus on the air entering your body. Listen to it slowly fill your lungs. Stroke your belly. Imagine the air moving into your baby. Exhale, slowly blowing out all of the negative thoughts and stresses of the day.

Each time you breathe, you are filling your body with goodness and light.

End this exercise only when you feel calm and serene.

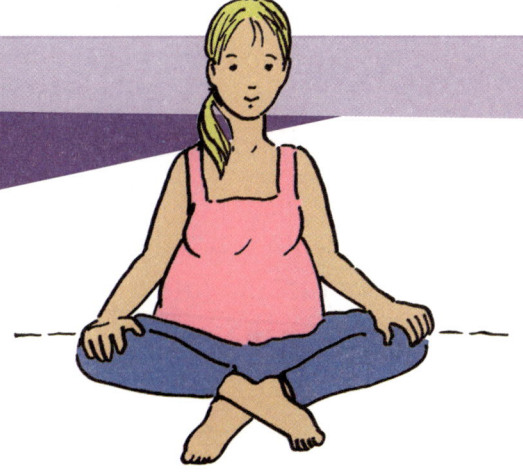

Many women who are pregnant find that writing in a personal journal every day gives them a needed outlet for their thoughts and feelings at this exciting time. A journal also is a place for women to record the changes they go through and the new experiences they encounter during their pregnancy. And not only does a journal "always listen to you," but in later years, you and your child will be able to look back and remember all the good things you did to make your baby's journey to this world the safest and most loving trip possible.

You have a group of muscles that essentially control your urine flow when you go to the bathroom. Pregnancy can stretch them and make incontinence (leaking urine) an unpleasant fact of life.

Kegel exercises strengthen the muscles that surround our pelvic region. These exercises are often talked about as an elevator ride—going up and down floors while tightening and releasing. As amusing as this game can be, it serves an important purpose: to make sure you do not have any embarrassing accidents now or in the future. You can practice this exercise in a chair, while waiting for a bus, sitting at a desk—anywhere. And no one will know you are doing it.

Kegel Exercise

You can tone the muscles that control urine flow. Here's how:

1. Sit comfortably in a chair and visualize the figure-8 shaped muscles that circle the vaginal opening and rectum along the pelvic floor.
2. Now tighten the area slowly, as if you are trying not to go to the bathroom.
3. Hold for about 5 seconds and then tighten some more.
4. Again, hold for another 5 seconds and then slowly release the muscles.

Educators liken this "tightening and releasing" to an elevator ride from the basement of a building to the top floor.

Do at least 10 of these "rides," tightening and releasing, three times a day for a good workout.

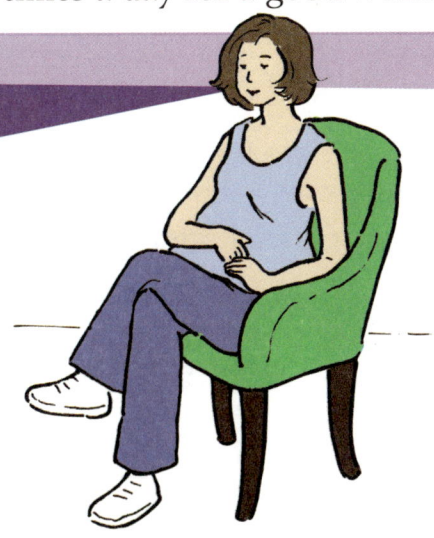

As enjoyable as a hot bath is, long hot baths and saunas are *not* advised during early pregnancy. Increasing your body temperature at such a sensitive time can potentially disrupt your baby's development and cause growth problems.

Find other good ways to relax. For example, after a quick shower, wrap yourself in a fluffy robe, sip your favorite herbal tea, listen to lovely music or read in a quiet room. Soak your feet in a basin of warm water that has been scented with rose water or lavender bath salts.

Do not put any substances into your birth canal—no douches or feminine hygiene products. Any of these can hinder, not help, your health by possibly reducing your birth canal's natural defenses against germs. Your body knows how to defend itself and your baby. It's best to leave it alone.

Imagine, about 20 years ago, pregnant women were advised—no, instructed—to gain only about 20 pounds during their pregnancy. This preposterously low number has inched up over the years. Today it is recommended that women gain 25 to 35 pounds over the course of their pregnancy.

The goal of nutrition during pregnancy is to keep you healthy and enhance your baby's growth. Worrying about gaining two pounds here and five pounds there is not productive. Where your eating is concerned, think long-term, not short-term: Think of delivering the healthiest baby possible!

As your pregnancy continues and the months pass, continue to focus your energy on eating healthful, nutritious food. Do not obsess about your weight! Give that job to your practitioner—if that makes him or her feel happy. As long as you feel well, and your baby is doing well, what's in a number?

Some moms are instructed to rest completely during pregnancy because of a medical condition or complication. This prescription often translates to mean *bed rest*. If you are on bed rest, try to fill your days reading books, chatting with friends, and doing light stretches to keep your blood circulating. Make it your top priority to reduce the risk that confined you to bed in the first place.

Bed rest is psychologically straining, but worth all of the pressure when your beautiful baby is born as healthy and strong as possible.

Contact your doctor or midwife about what type of exercises, foods and activities are suitable for a bed-resting mom. Remember, he or she wants you to have a healthy baby, too.

Your practitioner knows all of the challenges a childbearing mother 40 years or older may face. While this information is helpful and important, it neither defines your own particular pregnancy nor guarantees that anything will happen to you or your baby.

It's true that some practitioners consider pregnant women more than 40 years old to be "at risk" for complications. Being "at risk" often means nothing more than having more prenatal appointments and tests than the average mom-to-be.

Remember that you have the right to respectful and considerate prenatal care. If your practitioner has forgotten that fact, you are free to remind him or her by using your consumer power and moving your care to someone else.

Notes to Tell My Doctor or Midwife:

Buying for Baby

Psst—I'll tell you a secret: All of the potions, lotions and products made for babies are really made for parents. Babies *do not care* if their bath oil is derived from pure, organic bee pollen, for example.

They just want a dry bottom, lots of love and a full belly.

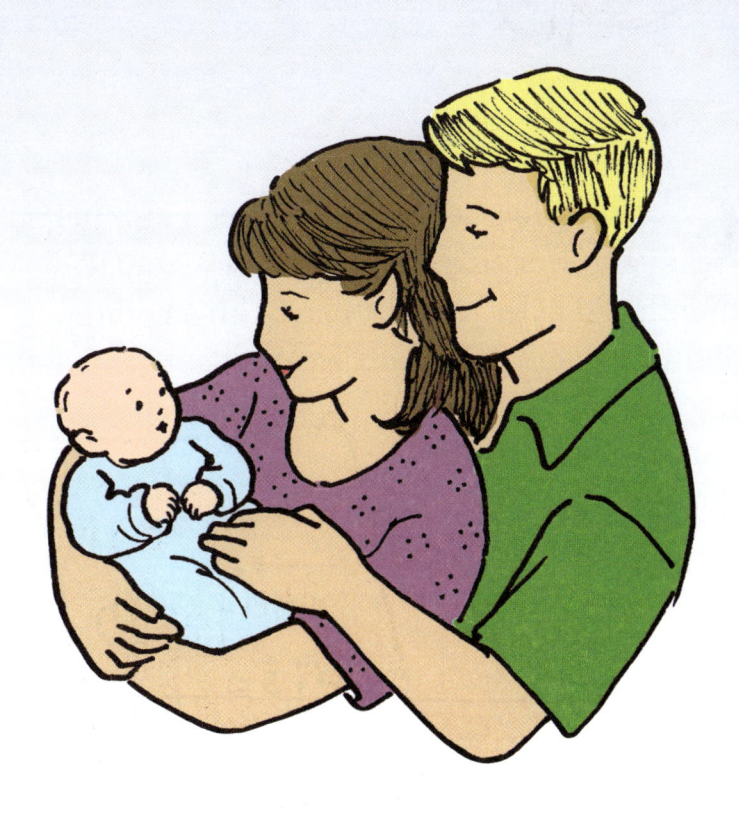

I t's tempting to purchase everything out there geared for babies, but try to resist. It helps to sit down and create a few lists before you go shopping. First consider what you know you need—such as a stroller and a car seat. Then jot down those things that would be nice to have. Finally, put down a few decadent luxuries—like a canopy crib or "theme"-pattern nursery wallpaper.

C reating lists of things you need also helps you prioritize baby purchases. Your 1-month-old baby will not play with a computer software game aimed at 2-year-olds. Resist that urge to buy one! Similarly, your baby due to be born in August won't need a snowsuit till next winter. Buy that item then.

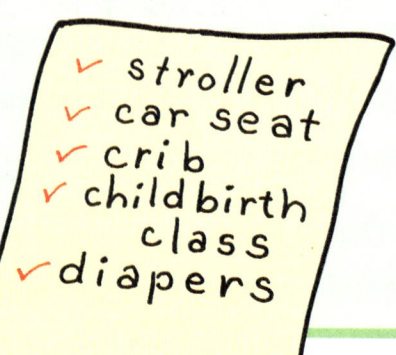

✓ stroller
✓ car seat
✓ crib
✓ childbirth class
✓ diapers

Active parents have many transportation options at their disposal. Today, you can buy an infant carrier that mom or dad wears like a front backpack. You can buy slings and rugged backpacks (once baby is older) too. You can find most of these products in a department store and in baby-gear mail-order catalogs.

Babies are legally required to ride in an infant car seat with approved safety features if they are in a moving vehicle. It is extremely important that you follow the manufacturer's instructions about connecting the infant seat to your car.

Many parents are confused by current instructions for installing the seats in their cars—it has been reported that up to 80 percent of these seats are installed incorrectly! That can have tragic consequences.

Take time to be sure you have installed the seat correctly. Don't be shy about asking for help if you aren't sure you have done it right. You can ask for help right at the hospital when you first take your baby home.

New Developments for Infant Car Seats

A new federal law requires all new cars and child safety seats to include an anchoring system that securely connects the baby seat to the car seat in several places. The requirements will be phased in over the next several years.

You don't automatically have to throw out an existing infant car seat you may have (provided you know it is in good condition otherwise, of course). Infant-seat manufacturers and car companies are offering kits for sale that address the safety concern.

The kits provide easy-to-use anchoring systems that will work in current car models and on existing infant car seats. The infant seat will attach better to the car seat with the modification. Eventually, all new infant car seats will come with the anchoring system incorporated into the seat design. And car companies will offer permanent infant-car-seat attachment points in all new models.

This is all good news for parents, because the anchoring system will make all the different car seats attach in the same way. If you have any questions about your car seat, contact the manufacturer. Concerns about your car can be addressed to the car company.

Any other questions about the law or the system can be directed to the National Highway Transportation Safety Administration at its web site: http://nhtsa.dot.gov or their hotline:

1 (800) DASH-2-DOT or 1 (800) 327-42368.

Infant car seats come in two varieties. One type is made for babies up to 20 pounds, and the other is designed to fit babies up to 40 pounds. Some car seats are designed for both.

Carriages and strollers have truly come full circle. Some of the most expensive "modern" carriages look exactly like the ones my mother-in-law used in England more than 30 years ago. They are high and bouncy—and are great for moms because you don't have to bend over so far to reach baby and pick him up. Even though the "new," color-coordinated carriages are fashionable, are they right for you? Ask yourself:

- ✿ Do I need a stroller that can handle outdoor trails?
- ✿ Or will I be walking mostly in the city on the sidewalk?

If you answer yes to the former question, a high, bouncy carriage style may not be right for your needs.

Jogging strollers are available for you moms who can't go without your daily exercise. Choose one with good straps to hold baby snugly in place.

Remember: Jogging strollers are not designed to be used on the roadway. Always jog with vigilance and good safety sense. You and your baby will enjoy the exercise more if you stay well away from automobiles and if you have taken all other safety precautions as well, such as using reflective tape or lights on your outfit and the jogging stroller (for high visibility).

A number of the nursery things available for purchase are pretty, but not necessarily helpful in caring for your baby. Before you buy, look around at all of your options. Ultimately you'll be happier with fewer items that give you more service than you would be with lots of "fun" items that just sit there, staring at you.

When you feel you are "at risk" of making an unnecessary baby purchase, pretend you are in a baby-store museum. . . . You are free to admire everything—but you don't take any of it home with you!

Some infant carriers on the market are intended for use only in the home. They often rock and enable baby to see everything around her. If you buy one, always check to make sure that your baby's seat is set up properly on a safe surface.

This Is Important

Never leave a baby unattended in any carrier on a counter or other high surface. Even if she is strapped in, her movements can move the carrier over the edge of the counter, causing a terrible fall.

You can find all kinds of infant swings. Some look like a park swing and move with the help of a spring. Other swings are fashioned more like a bed and rock mechanically. Use these sorts of products safely by following the manufacturer's instructions *every time* you use them.

As beautiful as crib sheets, bed skirts and pillows with streamers are to you, they pose a choking or strangling hazard to your baby. Keep them out of the crib, please.

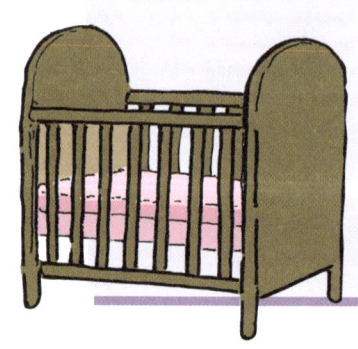

Keep your baby's bed uncluttered. Do not allow stuffed toys, ribbons or large blankets in baby's crib, either. All of these things can potentially cover baby's face and are suffocation hazards.

If you purchased your baby's crib from a secondhand store or received it from a friend, check it out thoroughly to make sure it is safe before you put baby in it. The spaces between slats on the side should not be big enough to allow baby's head to get trapped. Most cribs made in the 1980s and later are up to the current consumer codes.

Cloth diapers are not what they used to be. Today, you can find them in cool colors and jazzy designs with simple fasteners—from snaps to Velcro® fasteners.

Diaper services are amazing businesses that operate like fairy godmothers. They take away bags of dirty diapers and bring back beautiful, sterilized, clean ones—all for a weekly fee. Believe me, if you are committed to using cloth diapers, but not interested in the cleanup, this option will feel like true luxury.

Disposable diapers came onto the market decades ago and seem to many of us modern mamas like progress. But while the ease and convenience of disposable diapers can't be beat, the cost is staggering. You could spend a sizeable sum buying diapers until your baby is 3 years or older.

Nowadays, disposable diapers come in prints, with leak guards, leg protectors and other goodies to keep your baby dry. All of these "perfections" come with a price tag, so look around for the brand that meets your baby's *and* your pocketbook's needs. Don't hesitate to be critical. Ask yourself which of the added conveniences your baby really needs—and which she can do without.

A few disposable-diaper companies use natural products in place of the standard chemical absorbents as their filler material. If a natural diaper product interests you, check out the offerings at your local health-products store.

Most newborn babies will need 6 to 10 diaper changes a day—if not more. Buy enough diapers *before* the birth to last at least a few days. Otherwise, you'll find yourself making a few unwelcome, middle-of-the-night trips to the 24-hour store.

Your little bundle will only be (on average) 7 or 8 pounds, plus some ounces, at birth. Why am I reminding you of this? Because you can probably skip buying those cute outfits for 2-year-olds for now.

Watch out for baby clothes that have cumbersome ties, strings, and snaps that you will have to undo and then redo every time you change your baby. Look for baby clothes that keep ties, strings and snaps to a minimum.

If your baby is born in the summer, try to limit his or her clothes to undershirts, gowns and sleepers that would fit a newborn- to 2-month-old. If your sweet baby will make a winter appearance, add hats, mittens, sweaters, snowsuits and thick blankets to your shopping and gifting list.

Even if you choose not to use cloth diapers on your baby, you still may want to purchase a dozen to keep on hand. They make excellent spill catchers and wipes.

A number of comforting groups exist to help breastfeeding mothers. One of the best known is La Leche League. You can contact them in the United States at 1(800) 525-3245, and in Canada at 1(613) 448-1842, for referrals to support groups in your area. La Leche League is devoted to supporting mothers who breastfeed or who want to breastfeed but need some extra help to get started. There is no fee for this. You are welcome to attend meetings and start learning about breastfeeding before you have your baby. Children are welcome at all meetings, too.

Circumstances sometimes make it necessary for a mom to try bottle-feeding her baby formula. If this is your situation, always follow the manufacturer's instructions about mixing or making the formula, and only put the formula into sterilized equipment.

Some dads feel left out of breastfeeding moments. But they don't have to be. Nurse near dad or share other duties with him—such as dressing, bathing or changing baby. Everyone in the family should feel involved in the caring for and loving of the new baby.

A newborn baby can recognize its mother's voice, while a new mother can identify her baby's cries. This "double imprinting" is one of the ways that both of you become attached to each other.

You will have to make a major decision before the delivery about where your baby will sleep. You have many options, from a co-sleeping arrangement to baby's own room.

Before you make any decisions, ask yourself these questions:

- ❀ How do I want to manage my nighttime duties?
- ❀ Where will baby spend most of his or her time in the house?

Sometimes other creative options—such as a modified crib that attaches to most adult beds—will be the right choice for your family.

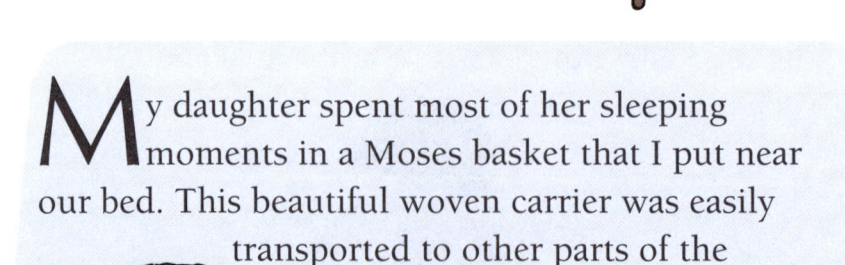

My daughter spent most of her sleeping moments in a Moses basket that I put near our bed. This beautiful woven carrier was easily transported to other parts of the house whenever I needed my little one to nap near me. Most major stores and plenty of specialty outlets carry this handy item.

Okay, you moms of multiples . . . listen up! You and your babies are strong and beautiful. Believe it! I want you (and them) to be one of the 50 percent of twin families who go to full term. Take care of yourself—eat well and sleep well. Pamper yourself whenever necessary.

Having more than one baby during one pregnancy can be exhausting *and* exhilarating. If this is your situation, seek information from lots of sources, and get help from friends and family! Talk to other mothers of multiples, read books and discover the Internet for practical ideas and support. Parenting more than one baby *is* doable, but you can't do it alone. Let others help you now, and know that down the road you'll do the same for someone else.

This might sound premature, but have you considered day care or even kindergarten for your baby? Amazingly, some cities have two-year waiting lists for day-care placement. If your long-term plans involve going back to work or school, check to see what the options are in your area soon.

If you are looking for a day-care situation, you must rigorously check out any caregiver you are considering. Get referrals to centers from mothers you trust. Then collect references from the centers and phone every one. Spend an entire day in the childcare center. Do everything you can to ensure that your little one is in the best possible hands in your absence.

Some people purchase expensive changing tables and then keep them in their baby's room far away on the second floor, even though they will spend most of their time downstairs during the day. This is absolutely silly and creates a lot of extra work for you, Mom! Your baby will want you to be a quick-change artist, so set up diapering areas (complete with supplies) throughout your home.

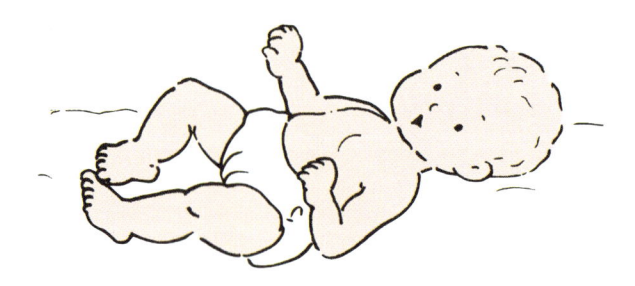

Tests and Special Concerns

Pregnancy is a perfectly natural occurrence. As in all other areas of life, however, difficulties can occur sometimes. If you are faced with any concern during your pregnancy—either to you or to your baby—seek help from one of the many resources that are available to you, locally or on the Internet. A number of support groups are included at the end of this book.

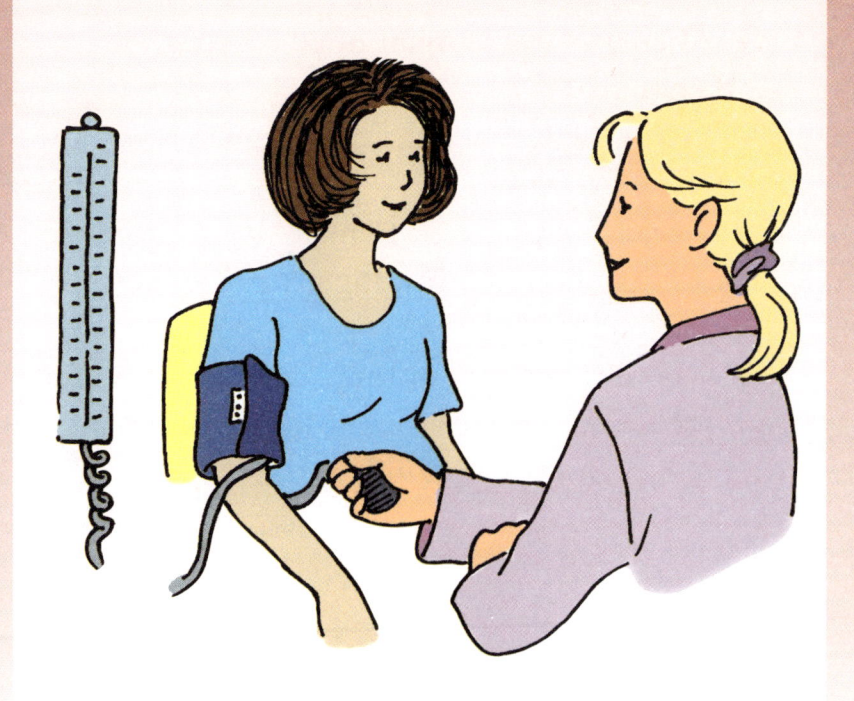

Most pregnant women today are faced with the challenging decision of taking or not taking various tests doctors use to check on a baby's condition. (Yes, you do have a choice!) The decision to take a test is challenging because it implies that still more decisions will have to be made after the results are in. Taking the test is not as important as what will be done with the results. Consider also that no test is 100% accurate; that fact can further complicate an already difficult situation.

When any test is mentioned by your practitioner, ask yourself:

❀ Would the test change my pregnancy or how I view my baby?

❀ Would I be prepared to make some difficult choices about continuing my pregnancy based on the results?

Your honest answers to these questions will tell you more about your attitude toward testing than a simple brochure ever could.

A few practitioners explain tests in a rush, without giving much background information—such as the risks it may pose to your baby. If you encounter a person like this, *ask again and again for more information* before agreeing to anything. It's your right to get the information you need for this important decision. Go to other sources for this information if you need to. Genetic counselors and web pages devoted to pregnancy issues are two sources that can supply the facts you need.

B e prepared to have your blood drawn at your first prenatal visit. It is usually tested for many routine things such as HIV—the human immunodeficiency virus. Ask that all test results be reported to you so that you are completely up-to-date about your and your baby's health.

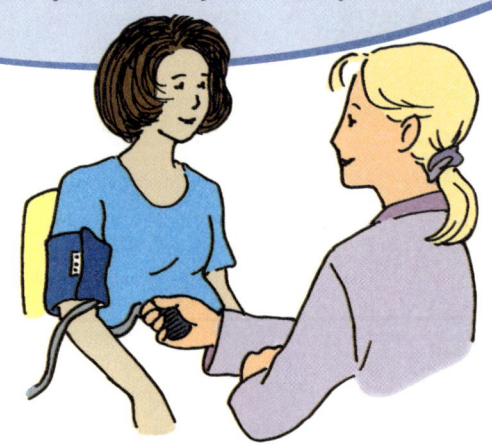

Do you remember if you had chickenpox as a child? Most of us can remember the itchiness of chickenpox and how long the illness seemed to last. If not, you might want to have your blood checked for its antibodies by your practitioner.

Your baby is protected from chickenpox exposure if you have had it in the past. If you haven't had chickenpox, you want to avoid getting it during pregnancy. Babies are not protected without mom's antibodies, and are at increased risk for birth defects if exposed early in the pregnancy, and other problems can occur if exposure occurs just before the birth.

If you are exposed to illnesses such as measles, mumps, fifth disease or rubella (German measles), tell your doctor or midwife immediately. You may only get mildly sick if you've never been exposed to the illness before. However, your baby may become quite sick. Always take exposure risks seriously. Miscarriages, birth defects, hearing loss and eye problems are some of the problems associated with exposure to these illnesses.

Many people confuse gestational diabetes with diabetes milletus (juvenile diabetes and Type II or adult-onset diabetes). Some of the complications involved are similar, but gestational diabetes is a rare occurrence that strikes a small percentage of women during pregnancy only. For most women, the condition goes away completely after the birth.

The hormones of pregnancy naturally suppress the body's production of insulin, a natural blood-sugar monitor. When insulin production is suppressed by the pregnancy, most women carry more sugar in their blood. The body uses this extra sugar to feed the baby in utero. In a few women, insulin suppression is so extreme that the baby gains a lot of extra weight because he receives the extra sugar in mom's blood. If you develop gestational diabetes, your practitioner will monitor you carefully so you can avoid this complication.

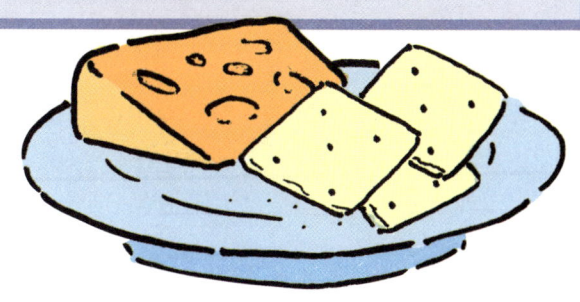

Don't Skip Prenatal Appointments!

Agood reason not to miss any of your prenatal appointments is the fact that they provide your doctor or midwife with an opportunity to diagnose and treat complications at an early stage, before they can do your baby or you any harm. Complications that typically can be caught early at prenatal appointments include gestational diabetes, high blood pressure, vaginal bleeding, breech presentation and urinary-tract infections.

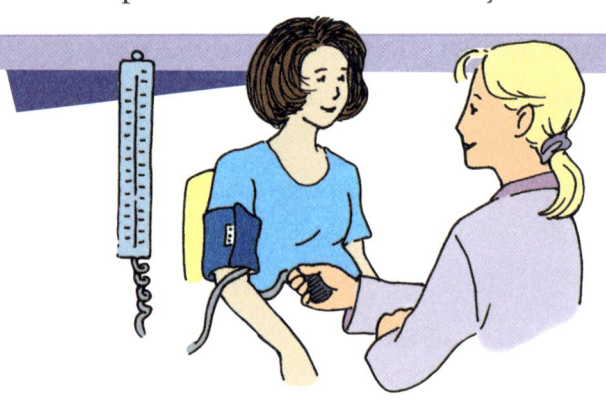

Mothers with an untreated diabetes mellitus condition frequently have exceptionally large babies who are at risk for a host of complications—from premature birth to respiratory problems. Because of the similarity of symptoms between gestational diabetes and regular diabetes, all pregnant women are encouraged to take a glucose tolerance test (GTT).

The glucose tolerance test is usually done between weeks 24 and 28 of pregnancy. It involves drinking an excessively sweet liquid called *glucola*. Mom's blood sugar level is measured about one hour after consumption to see how her body responds to the added glucose or sugar.

If the results from a 1-hour glucose tolerance test come back reflecting high levels of sugar, a 3-hour test is usually recommended next. If mom gets a second positive result from this test, she may have to go on a special diabetic diet. Talk with your practitioner about this so that you are well informed about the most current research and recommendations.

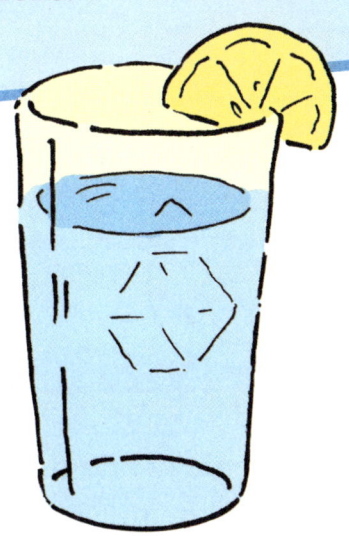

Toxoplasmosis is a condition caused by a parasite found in undercooked meat or in cat feces. Most people have been exposed, but if you haven't, your baby can get quite sick from it— fever, jaundice and premature delivery are all potential problems. How can you prevent it?

1. Make sure all meat is well cooked.
2. Scrub kitchen counters with cleanser to remove any raw-meat juices. Also carefully wash cutting boards and utensils in hot, soapy water if they have been in contact with raw meat.
3. If you have a cat, give it only store-bought food. (Mice can harbor the parasite.)
4. Have someone else clean the litter box.

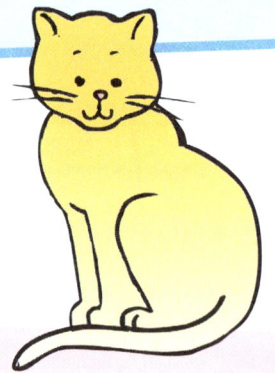

Always question your practitioner about the need, the benefits and the risks of a test so that you can make the most informed decision about your care.

When someone's iron levels are too low, he or she is said to be *anemic*. Symptoms of anemia include fatigue and tired muscles. (Sounds like pregnancy, right?) A finger-prick test at a prenatal visit can measure the hematocrit and hemoglobin levels of your blood. These levels tell your healthcare practitioner if you have normal iron levels, or are borderline or fully anemic.

Anemic mothers are at increased risk for delivering a premature or low-birthweight baby. Once you know your status, talk to your practitioner about whether you need to adjust your diet to include more iron, or take an iron supplement.

Remember, as beneficial as iron supplements can be, they have a tendency to slow down your natural disposal system, causing constipation. Want some surefire remedies?

1. Eat high-fiber foods (see page 25).
2. Walk—Walking is like a massage for your intestines. It keeps stuff moving!
3. Drink plenty of water. Think of it as flushing out the system.

Pre-eclampsia is a condition that typically occurs late in pregnancy. Very few women actually develop pre-eclampsia, but the screening is necessary for all women because symptoms can come on suddenly. It includes a variety of symptoms—protein in the urine, high blood pressure, swollen limbs and headaches. Untreated, it could affect mom's health and the growth of her baby.

Pre-eclampsia can range from mild to severe. If any of the signs are present—see previous tip—your doctor or midwife will monitor you closely.

Pre-eclampsia is often treated with bed rest. In severe cases, a practitioner may prescribe medications for the pregnant woman to reduce her blood pressure, or an early delivery of the baby may be recommended. Talk to your practitioner at length about this condition so that you are aware of all the events that could unfold before they do.

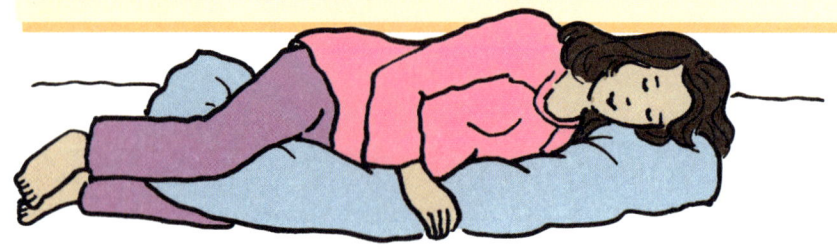

Babies produce a substance in their livers called *alpha-fetoprotein* (AFP). This substance can be measured in mom's blood from a sample taken from her arm.

The alpha-fetoprotein screening test, done between weeks 16 and 18, is an important risk marker for determining potential problems or concerns for a baby's health. Low levels of AFP indicate a possible chromosomal defect, such as Down syndrome. High levels indicate a possible problem in or around the spinal cord, such as spina bifida.

The alpha-fetoprotein screen carries no physical risk to mother or baby, but can cause a lot of psychological stress to parents, given that the results often lead to more tests.

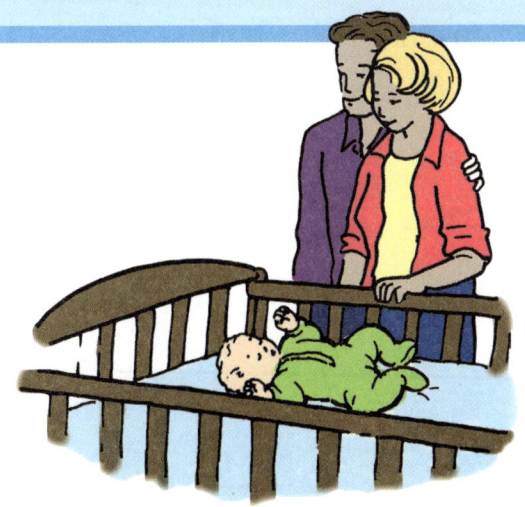

Amniocentesis is a test that evaluates a baby's chromosomes. This genetic test is usually done between the twelfth and sixteenth week of pregnancy. It involves inserting a needle into the womb (avoiding baby and the placenta) to gather a sample of amniotic fluid (the water-like fluid surrounding baby in the uterus).

Doctors use ultrasound to look inside the uterus using high-frequency sound waves. A small, hand-held device sends the waves into the womb. The waves bounce off tissue and create an image by covering an entire area; in this case, your uterus.

The image or picture is displayed on a small television-like screen. Displayed there is your baby! You can see his hands, his mouth, his arms, feet and legs, his fast-beating heart and other organs, and you can even tell his sex.

An ultrasound is used for many diagnostic purposes—for example, to determine the age of the growing baby in the womb, to check on developing organs in the baby and even to spot any physical abnormalities.

An ultrasound scan is used to guide the needle safely in its quest for fluid during an amniocentesis. Even with that kind of care, this particular test does rarely cause a miscarriage. The number of mothers who are affected are low (about 1 in 200), but you should be prepared to take this risk before you agree to the test.

The amniotic fluid gathered in an amniocentesis is taken to a lab, where it is essentially shaken and stirred to reveal the baby's genetic makeup. This test reveals the baby's unique chromosomal patterns, any abnormalities—and also its sex.

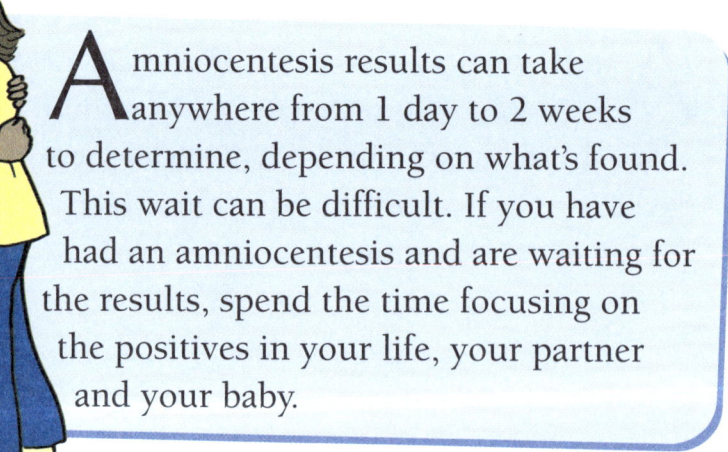

Amniocentesis results can take anywhere from 1 day to 2 weeks to determine, depending on what's found. This wait can be difficult. If you have had an amniocentesis and are waiting for the results, spend the time focusing on the positives in your life, your partner and your baby.

You may have heard about a special test called *chorionic villus sampling*, or CVS. CVS is a chromosomal test done earlier in pregnancy than an amniocentesis—around weeks 8 to 12. This earlier time frame comes at a price—the risk of miscarriage is higher for this test than it is for an amniocentesis; about 1 in 100 women will miscarry because of the CVS test.

A chorionic villus sampling test involves taking a sample of the finger-like hairs that surround the baby early in pregnancy.

Parents weigh the decision of having chorionic villus sampling carefully. These are some factors to consider:

- ❀ Make sure that you are well informed about your baby's risk of chromosomal abnormalities before you agree to it.
- ❀ Think about what you plan to do with any results you receive, positive or negative.
- ❀ If you would not change a thing about your pregnancy regardless of the test results, ask yourself why you might want to take the test.

Sometimes, for no apparent reason, a pregnancy just doesn't continue and a baby is lost. This is *very* tough, of course. It doesn't matter if the pregnancy was 3 weeks or 4 months along—that is a life to grieve. Seek help from counseling and support services to get through this difficult time.

Chromosomal tests are routinely advised for women 35 or older because they are more likely to have problems with egg abnormalities. If you are older than 35, ask yourself some important questions about your baby, this pregnancy and future pregnancies before agreeing to any tests. Some questions you might ask yourself are:

1. Will this be my only pregnancy?
2. Would I continue with the pregnancy no matter the diagnosis?
3. Is the risk of the test worth the benefits?

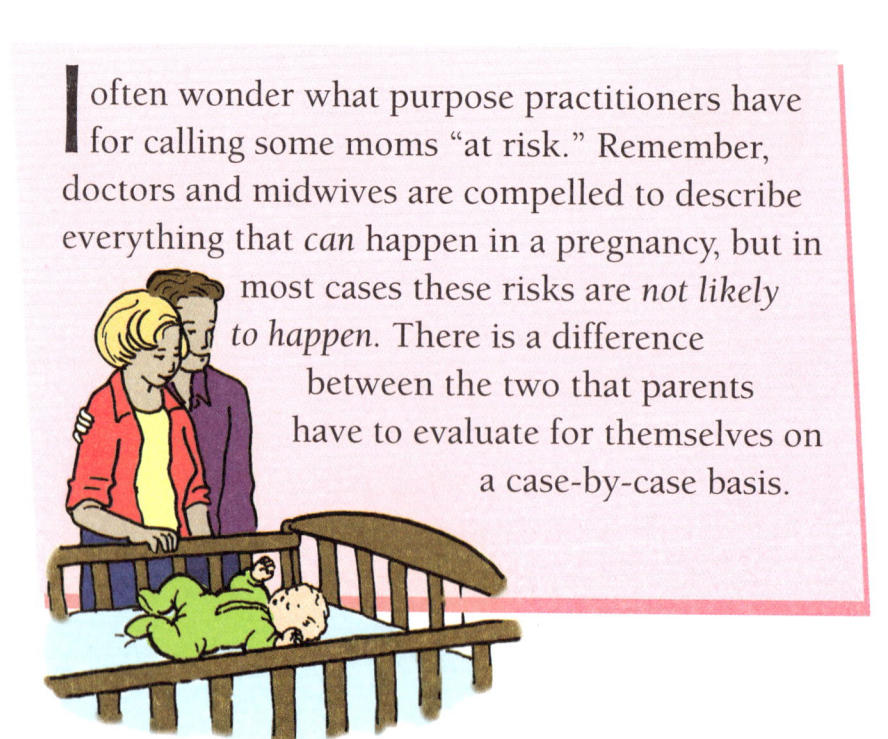

I often wonder what purpose practitioners have for calling some moms "at risk." Remember, doctors and midwives are compelled to describe everything that *can* happen in a pregnancy, but in most cases these risks are *not likely to happen.* There is a difference between the two that parents have to evaluate for themselves on a case-by-case basis.

*G*roup B streptococcus (GBS) is the long name for a common bacteria that most women have in their vagina. Although they sound similar, this is a different type of *streptococcus* bacteria than the one that causes the illness known as *strep throat*.

As common as group B streptococcus is, it is a bacteria that can give baby a serious infection if he or she is exposed to it. A simple culture swab from your vagina alerts your practitioner to the presence or absence of this bacteria.

Group B streptococcus is treated with antibiotics. If you are in labor and GBS is suspected, you will be given intravenous antibiotics.

*C*ontroversy surrounds the testing for Group B streptococcus. Some practitioners feel that the risk of infection is high enough to give every mother antibiotics during labor to combat it. Other practitioners believe that most mothers aren't at risk, and those who are can receive false-negative results because the culture test is often inconclusive. Talk to your practitioner about his or her feelings about this test well before your due date if it concerns you.

Your doctor or midwife wants you to be healthy throughout your pregnancy and the delivery of your baby. If medication or tests are recommended, you need to know exactly why your practitioner wants you to take the medication or the test and its effect on you and your baby. Don't ever be afraid to ask the questions that are on your mind.

You and
Your Partner

It's often difficult to put into words to your partner the amazing changes that are going on inside you. But for his involvement and growth as a dad, try to share. Your relationship will benefit from starting out the pregnancy as a team.

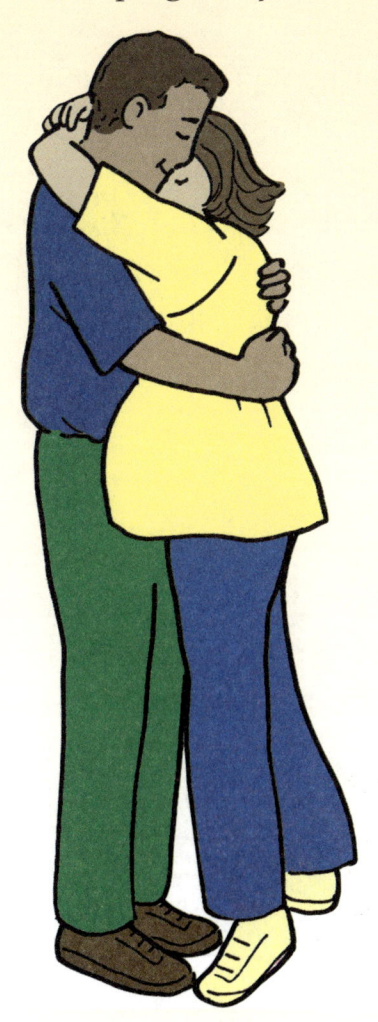

Some men have been conditioned to believe that pregnant women are something other than sexy, vibrant and gorgeous. If your man sometimes forgets how incredible you are, do something to remind him why he fell in love with you in the first place.

No matter how you feel about having a baby—scared, happy, stressed— your partner needs to share your emotional ride. Besides, he might be feeling the same way. Remember, there's no blueprint for being a terrific partner in pregnancy. Show and tell him what helps you.

It's kind of hard to be loving and passionate when all you can think about is trying not to throw up. Try to lessen your trauma by ridding your home of things that make you feel sick. This may mean certain foods or smells are outlawed in your house!

Few things are as magical as the first time you feel your baby move inside of you. Share the kicks of your budding soccer player with your partner. Have him put his hands against you so that he too can feel this miracle of life.

One exercise I recommend for couples in my childbirth classes is what I call *the double belly rub*. Mom sits comfortably on the floor with dad behind, supporting her back. Together, mom and dad gently caress the life they created. Most babies love it, and respond by kicking, as if to say, *Hello, I'm here*.

There will probably be times during your pregnancy when the old spark just isn't there. For reasons that may be unknown to you, the sexual urge vanishes. If it happens, remember that while it may be frustrating for you, it could be downright spooky for your man. Make sure he knows that you have not lost interest in him, that you still love him dearly, but that you might need a few more cuddles instead of sex right now.

Sometimes a massage in all the right places is just what you need to feel loved again. Let your partner know what you need and see what happens!

Believe it or not, some women feel more sexual during pregnancy than ever before. Perhaps the extra blood flowing through the body is helping them to feel what some mothers have called *ecstasy*.

One of the most common misguided beliefs about sex during pregnancy is that the act itself will harm the baby. This is not true unless some other concern such as preterm labor, infections or placenta problems are suspected or have already been detected. The strong muscle that surrounds the baby, called the *uterus*, protects it from harm during sex.

If you feel burning, stinging, or painful sensations during lovemaking, stop immediately. Contact your practitioner for a visit to check things out. Sex should not be painful.

Some Relationship Must-Haves during Pregnancy

Candles—Light them everywhere. Choose scented ones if you enjoy that. Lavender scents enhance relaxation.

Oils—For the bath and the body. Massage, anyone?

Cuddles—Lots of these. Even with your bounteous belly, you need to feel your man's arms around you.

Long walks together—Long is relative here, because you might only make it down the block and back during your last weeks of pregnancy.

Quiet time—Light a fire and sit together just staring at the flames and each other. If it's too hot where you live, perhaps you might choose to watch a setting sun or listen to waves lapping a lakefront or crashing against a beach.

Love—That essential ingredient. Focus on it. Treat it like a precious gem.

Prepare yourself and your partner for the inevitability of change; especially in the way your body will look. Unfortunately, in this country, many men are not used to seeing pregnant women as beautiful. So check out some books from the library, with tasteful pictures, to show him, and you, how lovely you will become.

Take time now, before your baby is born, to talk to your partner about your parenting goals and fears.

A few fathers have expressed to me their fear of not having enough money to rear their family in the way they would like. This may not describe your man, but if it does, take time to talk with him about his concerns. If you need to, consult an accountant about how best to budget your money in order to accomplish your financial goals.

My husband took weekly pictures of me during my first pregnancy. These beautiful images show the amazing changes that my body went through to develop my twin babies into 6-pounds, 9-ounces, and 7-pounds, 7-ounces of energy. You too might appreciate having some sort of pictorial account of this magical time.

It is possible during pregnancy to feel anxious, frightened, excited, tired, angry and sad about everything—even in the same hour! Sometimes your man may find himself at the receiving end of your distress. Try to sit down with him *before* you feel overwhelmed and explain your conflicting emotions. Men are smarter than we sometimes give them credit for. With a little specific information from you, he'll figure out how best to help you.

Disagreements between you and your partner may arise occasionally about how you will rear your baby. For sanity's sake, try to focus on your similarities instead of your differences in this area. Besides, as comforting as it may be to think that you are right, remember that no one yet has come up with a "perfect" formula for rearing kids. Parenting is shared learning at its best!

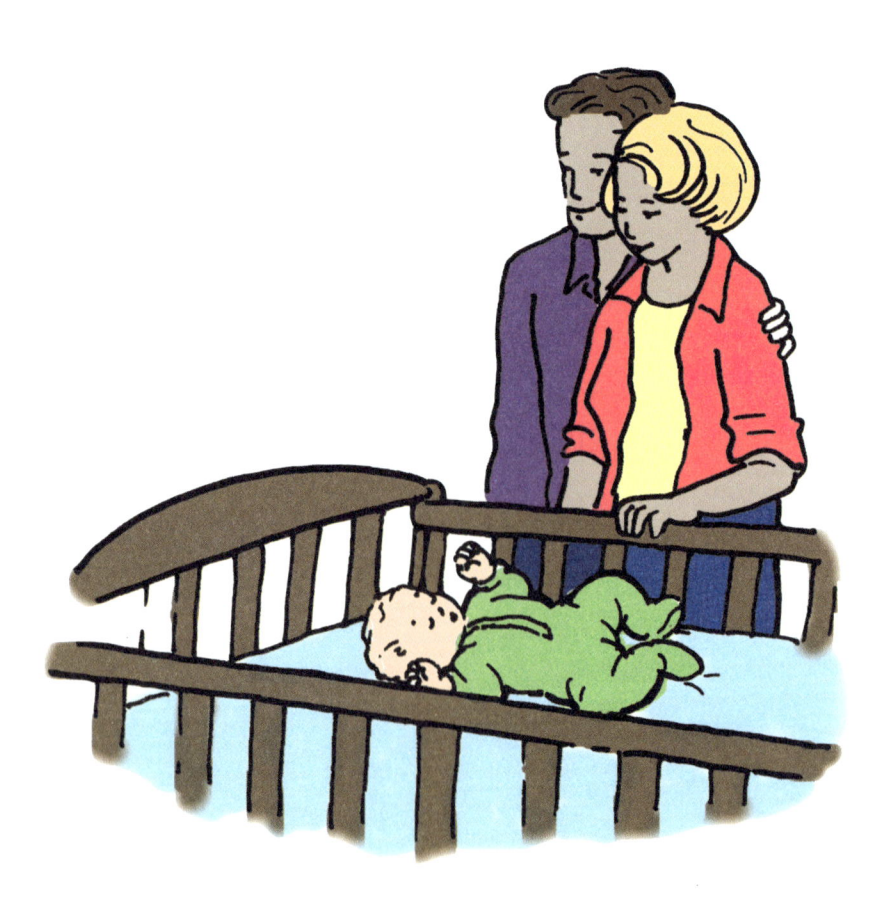

Preparing for Birth and Beyond

As your pregnancy progresses, you will naturally start thinking more and more about your due date and the delivery of your baby. A childbirth class is not only an important place to find knowledgeable and supportive friends, but also it is a great place to ask questions and learn about what happens in labor and delivery.

Early pregnancy, pre-pregnancy and postpartum classes are also available in many cities. It's best to sign up for childbirth classes sometime in your seventh or eighth month.

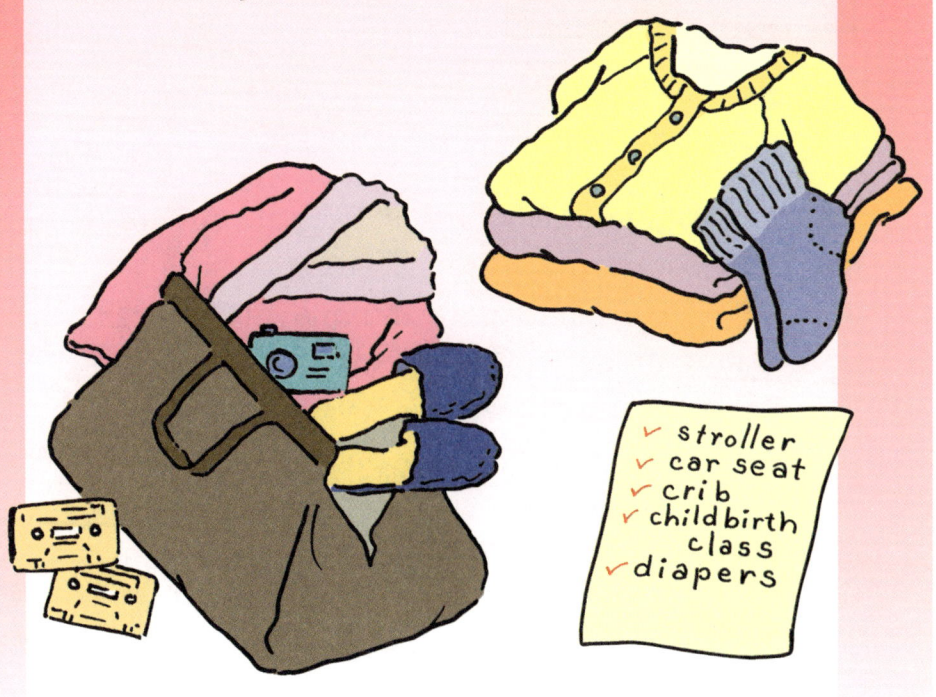

✓ stroller
✓ car seat
✓ crib
✓ childbirth class
✓ diapers

Childbirth educators come from a number of different groups—like Lamaze International, Birthworks, the Association of Labor Assistants and Childbirth Educators, the Bradley Method and the International Childbirth Education Association. Each group has a slightly different philosophy and may teach a slightly different birthing method, but they all believe that mothers, fathers and babies are beautiful.

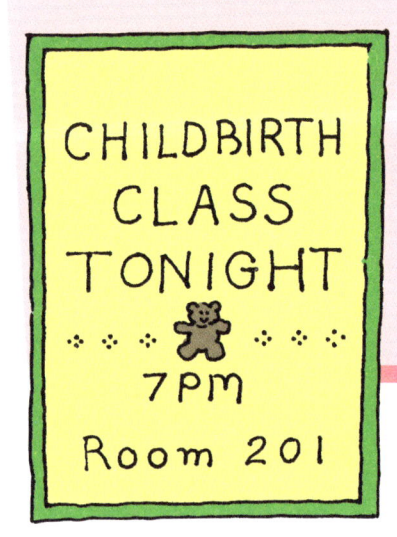

CHILDBIRTH CLASS TONIGHT

7PM

Room 201

You can find childbirth classes in your area by contacting hospitals, county health departments, and doctor's and midwife's offices. Your practitioner or a friend may be able to refer you to someone specifically. Ask around. If you are particularly interested in a certain type of class, contact friends or go on the Internet for referrals to qualified educators in your area.

As your due date approaches, your baby prepares to leave her temporary home. This temporary home inside of you is known by a number of different names: *uterus* and *womb* are two examples.

Your uterus is shaped like a hot-air balloon, with the basket part protruding into your birth canal. What's most amazing about a woman's uterus is that it expands to accommodate a growing bundle of joy.

The bottom part of your uterus is called the *cervix*. It can be felt at the end of your birth canal. When your practitioner talks about *effacement* and *dilation*, he or she is talking about changes to your cervix that need to happen before your baby can be born.

Babies develop their most-needed friend in the first few weeks of pregnancy: the placenta. This large, disc-like organ works as baby's stomach, lungs, arteries, veins, liver and rectum. It is also involved in keeping the pregnancy going.

The placenta is the organ that connects mom and baby. The umbilical cord—the twisted artery-and-vein "rope" connected to baby—attaches to one side of the placenta. The other side of the placenta is attached to mom through blood vessels that more or less burrow into her uterus.

Your baby lies nestled inside your warm uterus in what some call *a bag of waters*. This "water" isn't water at all. It's a salty, protein-and-nutrient-packed solution that protects baby against infection.

Your practitioner calls your bag of waters *amniotic fluid*. This fluid does not appear until about the fourth week of your pregnancy. You and your baby eventually will produce this fluid together.

A bag holds in the amniotic fluid that surrounds the baby in the womb, and it is actually composed of two membranes known as the *chorion* and the *amnion*. Most people just discuss the amnion. Once your baby is born and the placenta comes out, you will have an opportunity to see the amnion. It looks like a clear, thin bag attached to the placenta.

Your baby in pregnancy is protected not only by the amnion, uterus and amniotic fluid, but also by what is known as the *mucous plug*. This plug (a glob of stringy mucus) is embedded in the center of your cervix. This plug comes out as the cervix starts to open—before or during labor.

When the mucous plug comes out of the cervix, you may notice pink stains in it. This pink color is blood from torn capillaries, which are our tiniest blood vessels. Capillaries surround the mucous plug in the cervix, and once it frees itself, they can be broken. Don't worry about the pink color or this tearing—it is a completely normal part of labor.

Labor usually starts soon after your mucous plug comes out—although some moms have gone a week after losing a mucous plug before having their first contraction.

Many women fear finding themselves in line at the bank when their water breaks. This is probably not likely. First, few women's water breaks before labor starts. And interestingly, those that do rupture are most likely to do so at night—*after* the banks are closed.

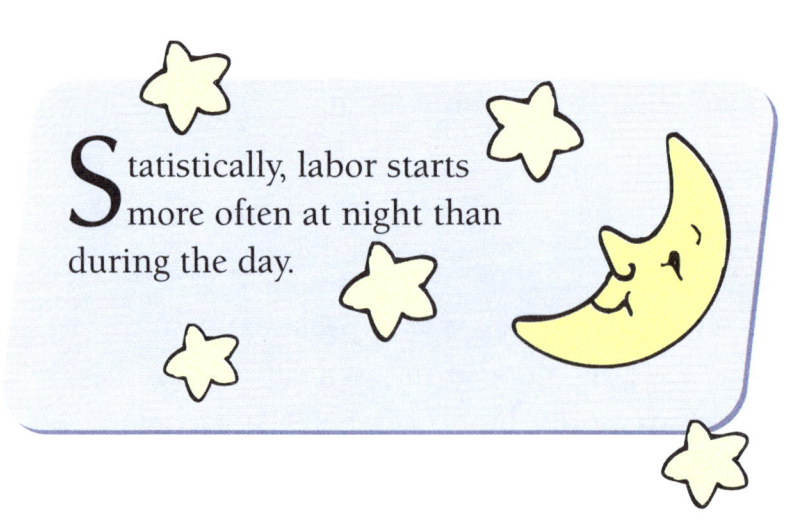

Statistically, labor starts more often at night than during the day.

When your "water breaks," you may notice a "pop" sound, followed by a gush or stream of warm liquid. This liquid, which is amniotic fluid, will continue to come out during labor because the body replenishes it constantly. So, wear cotton pads in your underwear to catch it—and change the pads often.

If your water breaks early, before labor starts, contact your doctor or midwife. He or she will most likely recommend that you not put anything inside your birth canal. Without the mucous plug to protect it, your uterus is at greater risk of infection.

Most women do not notice that they are in early labor until their contractions start coming in some kind of pattern.

During a contraction, the top of your uterus tightens (along with your abdominal muscles) into a hard ball. What's interesting is that the lower part of your uterus relaxes at the same time! The tightening at the top enables the lower band of the uterus, called the *cervix,* to be pulled open. And because the cervix needs to open for your baby to be born, this is a good thing.

Your practitioner may have already talked to you about contacting his or her office when your contractions are about 5 minutes apart. This number matters a great deal. So does your perception of the contractions. The pattern of the contractions will change gradually. The contractions at the beginning of labor may claim some of your attention, but typically they do not feel as intense as the contractions later, which bring about full dilation of the cervix.

How Will I Know if I'm in Labor?

Labor is different for every woman, but usually some pattern establishes itself. A mom in labor typically

1. Feels contractions that get stronger and closer together
2. Feels crampy and may have lower back pain
3. Feels excited or maybe a little nervous
4. Feels sensations in her cervix that may resemble tugging or pulling (This is the cervix shortening in length and opening to accommodate the baby's head.)
5. Feels contractions no matter what—even if she sits or goes to bed
6. Feels her contractions getting stronger when she walks around
7. Is beautiful and strong!

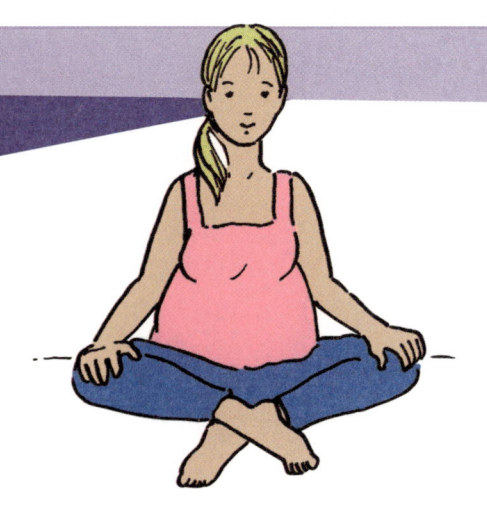

What Will My Labor REALLY Be Like?

I wish I could tell you. But I can't. Every woman is unique. Some mothers describe the pain of contractions as being a total, body-consuming thing, while others describe no pain at all! I can't say what the contractions will feel like to you, because so much depends on your pain threshold and your energy level before labor starts. Similarly, for some women, labor is long, and for others, it is short—very short. My best advice is for you to try to stay relaxed and let your body follow its course.

When your baby is born, whom do you want with you besides the father? Your sister? Mom? Your best friend? Ask yourself this question and answer it honestly. You do not want people who drive you crazy present at one of the most special moments in your and your baby's life.

An old, yet new, professional has appeared on the birth scene recently to help pregnant and birthing women and their families. This person goes by many names—*monitrice, professional labor assistant, doula, labor support person*, and even *birth assistant*.

Doulas or professional labor assistants are trained and often certified to support women during labor. They know positions that can speed labor along and decrease discomfort. They also tend to bring along hot packs, massage oils and other items to the delivery to help relieve mom's tension and promote relaxation.

Many doulas can be hired to appear just *after* baby is born. The goal of this postpartum support person is to help with feeding, guide infant care, and often just to help mom and the rest of the family get back on their feet after an exciting and exhausting event. Doulas free the new mother and the rest of the family to concentrate on bonding with the new baby.

Doulas principally believe that they are on the scene to "mother the mother" by giving her support and encouragement. They neither take over the birth as their own, nor force any decision on the mother.

If you are interested in finding a doula or labor assistant in your area, contact your doctor or midwife for referrals. National organizations such as Doulas of North America (Contact them on the Internet at www.dona.com) and the Association of Labor Assistants and Childbirth Educators (Call 1(888) 22-ALACE) can also provide you with a list of nearby professionals.

Studies show that having a doula during labor and birth can reduce a mom's need for a Cesarean, lower her epidural use, and increase her confidence in her parenting abilities.

Pregnant women today have a number of pregnancy and birth practitioners to choose from. Midwives, family practitioners, obstetricians, nurse practitioners and others all catch babies and guide mothers through an amazing year of change.

In many communities, birth centers, homebirth services and hospital maternity units all exist to offer mothers the opportunity to give birth where they feel the most comfortable.

If you want to deliver your baby at home or in a birth center, contact the providers of these services and interview them at length well ahead of time so that you are comfortable with every issue. You can also go on the Internet to find more information. Try these sites:
http://www.parentplace.com, and
http://www.parentsoup.com

ospitals today are remembering that pregnant women are giving birth when they arrive at the hospital, not having their tonsils removed. Gone in many places are standard "medical" practices that aren't crucial to a safe birth—such as shaving mom's pubic hair. Dads are in the birthing room—in large numbers. Believe it or not, some hospitals offer birth suites with cable, queen-sized beds and even gourmet meals!

Labor is the term used to describe an amazing event leading up to the birth of your baby. And it is an accurate description. Your body will have never worked this hard before!

As exhausting as labor can be, nothing can prepare you for the magical moment when your baby comes into the world. Your heart may swell with more love than you thought was possible the moment your bundle is in your arms. Some moms don't experience this rush. Instead they may feel scared or just overwhelmed. It's okay if you feel all of these different emotions. You and your baby have gone through an amazing event. Take the time to recover both your body and your senses.

What to Bring to the Birth

You have the option of bringing a number of items with you to your baby's birth.

🌸 **A favorite shirt or gown** to labor in is often a good idea.

🌸 **A robe**, in case you decide to stroll the halls.

🌸 **Socks or slippers** are must-haves for those cold floors.

Other things are more comfort-related:

🌸 **Music and a device to play it on**

🌸 **Favorite pictures**

🌸 **Massage oil**

🌸 **A personal phone book** and a calling card or lots of coins (your partner will want to spread the good news as soon as baby is born)

🌸 And don't forget **your camera**!

You will need more clothes for yourself after your baby's birth, including going-home clothes for you and your baby.

Labor technically comprises different stages known as the *first, second* and *third stages of labor*. These terms describe the changes your cervix goes through to bring your baby's head into your birth canal, your pushing efforts to bring baby out of your body, and the "birth" of the placenta, also called the *afterbirth*.

The first stage of labor is itself made up of three different phases.

Phase One   The early phase of labor is just that: the early changes. Labor is not considered active during the early phase.

Phase Two   Once active labor starts, when the cervix is 4 to 5 centimeters (cm) in dilation, things really start to pick up!

Phase Three   The last phase is the often-talked-about *transition time*, when the cervix goes from 8 to 10cm in dilation, and your baby is ready to be born.

Your cervix, the lower part of your uterus that's in the vagina, changes texture and shape to bring your baby into your birth canal. Practitioners use big words like *effacement* and *dilation* to describe this process.

Your cervix is thick and tightly closed before labor starts. Once labor begins (or just before), the cervix starts to thin, or *efface*—in much the same way that a thick rubber band thins out as you stretch it. This thinning allows *dilation* (the opening of the cervix) to occur with ease.

Your cervix is said to be *fully dilated* when it is 10 centimeters (cm) in diameter. This enables your baby's head to enter your birth canal.

The dilation of your cervix from 0 to 10cm can be very intense. Contractions get closer together, and last longer—and longer. Contractions essentially press your baby's head against your cervix, and pull the muscles at the opening of your cervix farther apart. Imagine pulling a tight turtleneck over your head. The stretching your head causes at the neck opening of the sweater is similar to the changes to your cervix during labor.

Timing contractions is not complicated, I promise. You simply write down the time at the start of one contraction, and then note the time at the *start* of the next one.

For example: You have a contraction at 10:10. It lasts for about 30 seconds. There is a pause, and then the next contraction starts at 10:17. You would note that your contractions are 7 minutes apart.

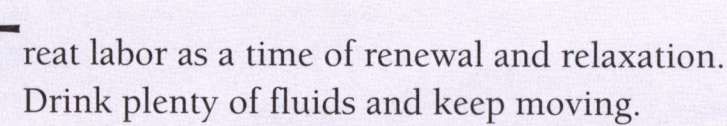

Treat labor as a time of renewal and relaxation. Drink plenty of fluids and keep moving. Equip yourself with relaxing music and your favorite comfort aids to help you get through this time with confidence and strength.

Back labor is an unpleasant reality for many women. What usually happens is that baby settles into a position that places immense pressure on mom's back. This pressure tends to linger between contractions.

How to cope? Massage, water and lots of support tend to help.

The good news: As if by magic, as soon as baby turns, the pressure disappears and the back pain vanishes.

Pushing a baby out of your body is a miraculous event. It is staggering what our bodies have been designed to do.

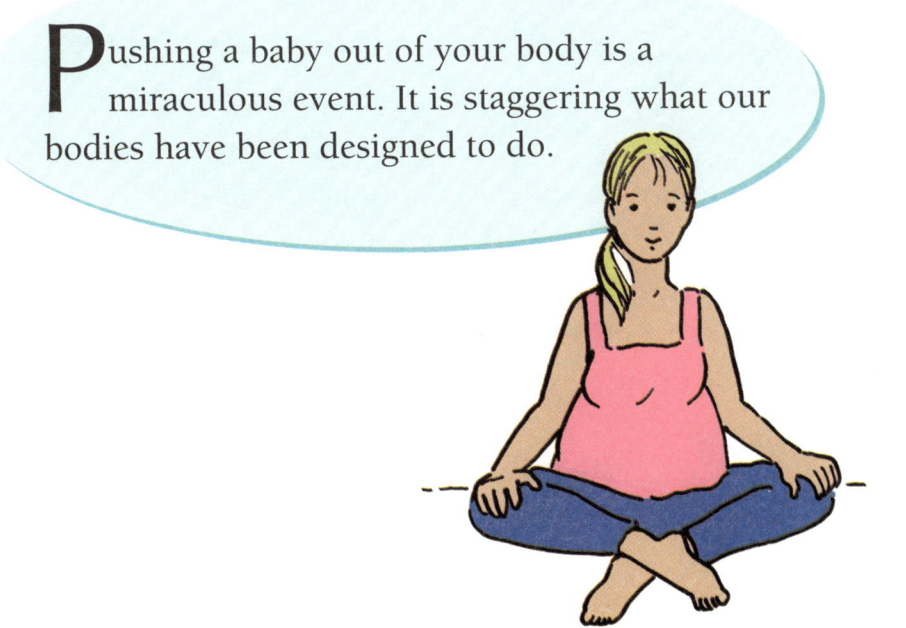

Use each contraction during the pushing stage to help guide your baby further down your birth canal. You can help make the pushing more effective.

Your uterus is squeezing your baby out with each contraction. As your baby's head pushes into your birth canal, she stimulates your automatic reflexes there that make you feel like pushing (as in "going-to-the-bathroom" pushing). Don't waste energy. Wait until the contraction starts and gets strong and *then* press your muscles (remember those Kegel exercises?) around your vagina toward the floor or the bed (depending on your position). Many health professionals recommend pressing intensely for a count of 10, then slowly relaxing. The pushing stage may last anywhere from 20 minutes to 2 hours or more.

You may have heard about an episiotomy from friends. It is a cut made by a doctor or midwife in the space between your vagina and your rectum. It is used to widen the vaginal opening during delivery.

Not every new mom needs an episiotomy. The area between the vagina and the rectum is elastic. It stretches to accommodate baby's head. In some instances, either baby's head is too big or birth needs to happen quickly and the doctor or midwife will choose to make this incision.

An episiotomy is a surgical incision that requires stitches to mend. You will need to recover from this procedure. Sitz baths—a small tub you can sit in with warm water—often relieve any discomfort.

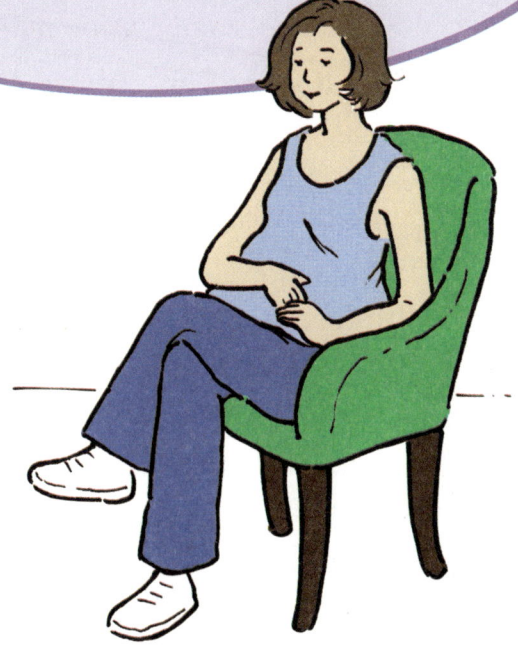

The Lowdown on Relieving Pain during Labor

Moms experience the "pains" of labor differently. Some feel uncomfortable in every spot of their body. Other moms feel intense sensations only as transition nears. Your experience may be the same or different.

No matter what you will experience, being as comfortable and as relaxed as possible is still your goal. With that aim in mind, I offer you a list of options that can relieve discomfort during labor. Please note that this list is not complete. Talk to your doctor, midwife or childbirth educator for more suggestions.

Water. A warm shower or soak in a tub can feel magical. *Good stress and tension relief.*

A tennis ball in a sock. This quick massage tool can be rubbed all over the back (avoid the spinal column). Many moms enjoy the pressure of the firm ball on areas that feel "tight." *Good tension relief.*

Comfort. A simple hug or stroke of the hand goes a long way toward making a mom feel supported. *Good stress relief.*

Wet cloths. Moms often find relief from a difficult contraction with the application of a cold coloth on the forehead or a warm cloth on the belly. *Good stress relief.*

Massage. Moms respond differently to massage. Some want only light stroking (or none); others want deep-tissue kneading (avoiding the spine). *May provide good tension relief.*

Positions. Sitting with, squatting next to and leaning on dad can change mom's perception of pain. *Good for enhancing labor; good pressure relief (especially during back labor).*

Scents. Candles or potpourri of relaxing scents can calm the soul. *Good relaxation device.*

Food. Labor can feel more difficult if the body does not have any energy. Water, juices, broth and toast are some early labor choices. *Good for enhancing labor.*

Analgesic drugs. These are medications, including nonprescription drugs such as aspirin, that relieve pain without loss of sensation or consciousness. A number of analgesics are available during labor. They affect mom and baby. *Partial or complete loss of pain. May be momentary.*

Anesthetic drugs. These are medications that bring about partial or complete loss of sensation, with or without loss of consciousness. *Epidural anesthesia* is an anesthetic. Again, this medication affects mom and baby. *Partial or complete loss of sensation.*

Note: Choose discomfort relief that matches your needs and enables you to continue to focus your energy on birthing your baby.

Circumstances beyond your control during your labor may require some sort of medical action or procedure. If you find yourself in this circumstance, be sure that you understand why the action is being considered and what procedures will need to be done as a result.

You may have heard from moms who have had a Cesarean section—about how frightening it is. Here's the truth: A Cesarean (also called a *C-section*) is a surgical procedure that involves cutting into the abdomen and the uterus to deliver a baby. It is major surgery, even though many women receive pain relief that removes all sensation, but keeps them awake. As with any major surgery, a recovery time is involved.

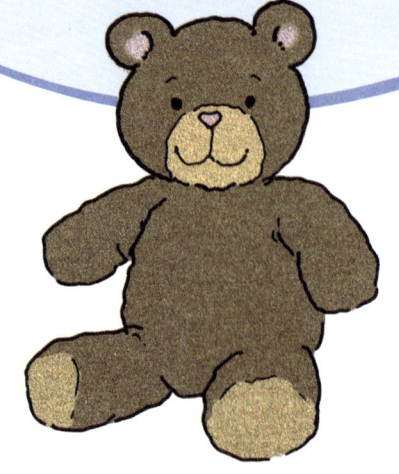

A Cesarean can be frightening, only because most women don't take the time to find out about this procedure and what is involved when they are still pregnant. Talk to your doctor or midwife now so that you are prepared for any eventuality.

Some mothers who have had a C-section report that they feel "cheated" of the birthing experience, and this makes them sad. If you need a Cesarean for any reason, remember: You are still a mother. You worked hard to get to the point of holding your baby in your arms. And you are working even harder now, to recover from your surgery. I recommend that you take time to reflect on your labor and the important reasons you needed to have a Cesarean. If you have been feeling sad about having a Cesarean, focusing on the positive reasons for having the surgery may help you feel better about your birth experience.

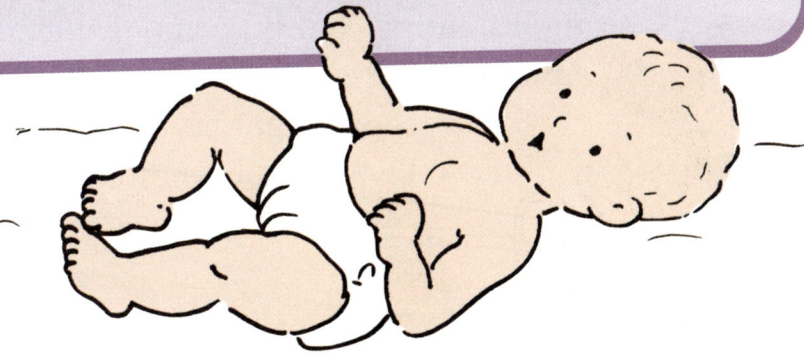

Many new moms now have their babies "room in" with them during their hospital stay. This option has become so popular that some hospitals no longer have a newborn nursery at all. Find out about this option at your local hospital.

As exciting as the entire nine months can be . . .

As transformational as labor and birth is . . .

None of this compares to the miracle that is now a part of your life. I have three of these miracles to behold every day. And my soul is richer because of them.

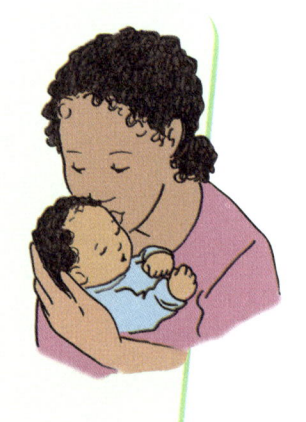

With your baby's birth, you may think that your journey is over, but it has only just begun. Parenting your little bundle into adulthood is truly a fantastic voyage. Some people might wish you good luck; I wish you good love.

Glossary

amnion. The innermost membrane of the sac containing amniotic fluid and the fetus during pregnancy.

amniotic fluid. The almost colorless fluid that surrounds the fetus in the amniotic sac, which protects the baby and helps maintain his temperature.

antibodies. Protein molecules created in the body that provide protection against certain foreign substances introduced into the body. Some antibodies can be transferred from mother to fetus during pregnancy.

bed rest. Prolonged rest in bed as treatment for a condition or illness. It can involve sporadic or complete periods of rest.

breech presentation. The baby may be in this position in the womb near or at birth. In this position, the baby's bottom comes out first, rather than its head.

Braxton Hicks contractions. Irregular, painless contractions that may occur after the third month of pregnancy. Toward the end of pregnancy, Braxton Hicks contractions increase in frequency. They do not represent a true sign of labor. Also called *practice contractions*.

cervix. The neck or opening of the uterus that protrudes into the vagina. It opens during birth to allow baby into the birth canal.

Cesarean section. Removal of the baby from the uterus by means of a surgical incision through the abdomen.

dilation. The expansion of the cervix during labor. It is measured from zero to ten centimeters in diameter. Ten centimeters is considered full dilation.

Doppler ultrasound. A hand-held device that changes sound waves into signals that are amplified by what looks like a small speaker. This device is used to hear a baby's heart tones. A Doppler ultrasound device can pick up a baby's heartbeat at or around the twelfth week of pregnancy.

edema. A condition in which fluids collect in certain body tissues and create swelling.

effacement. The thinning of the cervix.

epidural. The space between the spinal cord and the protective sheath covering it. An *epidural block* is a type of anesthesia that is injected into this space during labor. It removes sensation and pain in parts of the body.

episiotomy. A surgical procedure done between the vaginal area and the rectum that widens the opening through which the baby's head emerges during delivery. It may be done if that tissue is otherwise suspected to tear during delivery.

human chorionic gonadotropin. A hormone elevated during pregnancy that is checked in tests to confirm or deny a pregnancy.

hypertension. High blood pressure.

insulin. A hormone that is essential for the metabolism of blood sugar. Insulin helps to regulate a proper blood sugar level in the body. Inadequate insulin production (or none at all) causes diabetes mellitus.

mucous plug. The gummy "stopper" that seals the cervical opening to the uterus. Losing the mucous plug may or may not mean labor is imminent; labor may start in hours, *or* in a week or two.

ovulation. The periodic discharge of an egg from an ovary, which occurs on average midway through the monthly menstrual cycle. There is typically a three- or four-day period during which a woman can become pregnant.

placenta. The spongy, pancake-like structure attached to the uterus through which the fetus gets nourishment and stores its wastes. The placenta is attached to the baby by the umbilical cord.

practice contractions. See *Braxton Hicks contractions.*

pre-eclampsia. A serious condition that can occur during pregnancy. Symptoms include high blood pressure, headaches and swelling in the legs, feet and hands. This condition requires close monitoring by a doctor or other healthcare practitioner.

umbilical cord. The attachment connecting the baby to the placenta, which contains two arteries and one vein. The umbilical cord carries nourishment to the baby from the placenta and also takes away the baby's waste products.

urinary-tract infection. Infection of the urinary tract by bacteria. Urinary-tract infections are common during pregnancy and should be treated promptly by your doctor. Signs of a urinary-tract infection may include a burning sensation upon urination or the urge to urinate when you don't need to.

uterus. The muscular organ that holds the baby throughout pregnancy. Also called the *womb*.

varicose veins. Enlarged veins close to the surface of the skin. They may occur in many areas of the body but are most common in the legs. Varicose veins can be a consequence of pregnancy. They are sometimes painful and may require a doctor's attention.

womb. See *uterus*.

Resources

Breastfeeding

La Leche League International
1400 N. Meacham Rd.
Schaumberg, IL 60168-4079
800-LA-LECHE
Breastfeeding helpline: 900-448-7475
Web: lalecheleague.org

Hospital for Sick Children Breastfeeding Clinic
555 University Ave.
Toronto, Ontario Canada M5G 1X8

INFACT (Infant Feeding Action Coalition Canada)
10 Trinity Sq.
Toronto, Ontario Canada M5G 1B1
416-595-9819
Web: infactcanada.ca

International Lactation Consultants Association
201 Brown Ave.
Evanston, IL 60202-3601

Doulas

Doulas of North America
Web: dona.com

Special Needs

Parents Anonymous
675 W. Foothill Blvd., #220
Claremont, CA 91711
909-621-6184

The Cleft Palate Foundation
11218 Grandview Ave.
Pittsburgh, PA 15211
800-242-5338

National Down Syndrome Society
666 Broadway, #810
New York, NY 10012
800-221-4602
Web: ndss.org

*National Organization of Mothers of
Twins Clubs, Inc.*
PO Box 23188
Albuquerque, NM 87192-1188
800-243-2276
Web: nomotc.org

*SHARE National Office
St. Joseph's Health Center*
300 First Capitol Dr.
St. Charles, MO 63301-2893
800-821-6819
Web: nationalshareoffice.com
Help with prenatal and postnatal bereavement

Birthing Resources

Childbirth Practices
ICEA (International Childbirth Education
Association)
PO Box 20048
Minneapolis, MN 55420-0048
612-854-8660
Web: icea.org

Birth Works, Inc.
PO Box 2045
Medford, NJ 08055
888-TO-BIRTH
Web: birthworks.org

Lamaze International
1200 19th St., NW, Suite 300
Washington, DC 20036-2422
800-368-4404
Web: lamaze-childbirth.com

The Bradley Method
American Academy of Husband Coached Childbirth
Box 5224
Sherman Oaks, CA 91413-5224
800-4-A-BIRTH
Web: bradleybirth.com

Association of Labor Assistants and Childbirth
Educators
PO Box 382724
Cambridge, MA 02238
617-441-2500
Web: alacehq.hypermart.net

Internet Resources

5aday.com
Nutrition information and detailed site that is part of the national 5-a-day fruits-and-vegetables campaign.

nal.usda.gov/fnic
Site of the Food and Nutrition Information Center of the U.S. Department of Agriculture. Excellent nutritional information.

nhtsa.dot.gov
Car seat and child passenger information from the National Highway Traffic Safety Administration of the U.S. Department of Transportation. This department continues to update infant car seat and transportation information.

parentsplace.com
This site has good general parenting and pregnancy information.

parenthoodweb.com
This site is a general pregnancy-and-birth resource.

pregnancytoday.com
This site is part of a larger site devoted to preconception, pregnancy, birth, breastfeeding and parenting issues. It is unique in that it is written by parents (with visits by experts).

babycenter.com
This excellent site has many pregnancy and birth articles.

INDEX